Health Dynamics and Marginalised Communities

Health Dynamics and Marginalised Communities

Edited by

Mohammad Akram

RAWAT PUBLICATIONS

Jaipur • New Delhi • Bangalore • Mumbai • Hyderabad • Guwahati

ISBN 81-316-0079-3

Published by
Prem Rawat for **Rawat Publications**
Satyam Apts., Sector 3, Jawahar Nagar, Jaipur 302 004 (India)
Phone: 0141 265 1748 / 7006 Fax: 0141 265 1748
E-mail: info@rawatbooks.com
Website: www.rawatbooks.com

New Delhi Office
4858/24, Ansari Road, Daryaganj, New Delhi 110 002
Phone: 011-23263290

Also at Bangalore, Mumbai, Hyderabad and Guwahati

Typeset by Rawat Computers, Jaipur
Printed at Chaman Enterprises, New Delhi

Contents

Contributors

Akash Acharya, Centre for Social Studies, Surat.

Balveer Singh, Mohanlal Sukhadia University, Udaipur.

B.L. Nagda, Population Research Centre, Udaipur.

B.V. Babu, Regional Medical Research Centre, ICMR, Bhubaneswar.

Chakrapani Upadhyay, Bhupal Noble's Post Graduate College, Udaipur.

Mihir Desai, Editor, *Combat Law*, Mumbai.

Mohan Advani, Mohanlal Sukhadia University, Udaipur.

Mohammad Akram, Aligarh Muslim University, Aligarh.

Madhu Nagla, M.D. University, Rohtak.

N.K. Jha, Government Post Graduate College, Pratapgarh.

P.R. Sodani, Indian Institute of Health Management Research, Jaipur.

Sujata Krishnamurthi, Associate Editor, *Combat Law*, Mumbai.

Supriya Seth, Government Post Graduate College, Kota.

Tribhu Nath Dubey, Government Post Graduate College, Kota.

Vijay Kumar Yadavendu, Zakir Hussain Centre for Educational Study, JNU, New Delhi.

Vani Verma, Vogilal Pandya College, Simalwara.

Y.S. Kusuma, Centre for Community Medicine, AIIMS, New Delhi.

Introduction

The Universal Declaration of Human Rights established a breakthrough in 1948, by stating in Article 25, "Everyone has the right to a standard of living adequate for the health and well-being of himself and his family...." The Preamble to the World Health Organisation (WHO) Constitution also affirms that it is one of the fundamental rights of every human being to enjoy "the highest attainable standard of health". The concept of 'right to health' is a broad term which includes several rights, viz., right to medical care, right to responsibility for health, right to a healthy environment, right to food, right to procreate (artificial insemination included), right to not to procreate (family planning, sterilization, legal abortion), and rights of the deceased persons (determination of death, autopsies, organ removal).

Article 21 of the Constitution of India states, "No person shall be deprived of his life or personal liberty except through procedure established by law". Till the 1970s, by and large, the courts had interpreted 'life' literally, i.e., right to exist. It was in late 1970s onwards that an expanded meaning started to be given to the word 'life'. Over the years it has come to be accepted that life does not only mean biological existence but the life of a dignified human being with all its concomitant attributes. This would include a healthy environment, life skill, education, food, nutrition and effective health care facilities.

The concepts of health, disease and treatment are related to the social structures of communities. Every culture, irrespective of its simplicity or complexity, has its own system of beliefs and practices concerning health and disease and has also evolved its own system of treatment to combat disease. With the rise of modern nation-states having specific welfare agenda, public health has become an inalienable aspect of civic life. States having the essence of civil society are evolving or adopting a health system suitable to its own needs, all over the world.

Health care promotion has been an integral component of all national health and family welfare programmes. Health status of a population, and especially of the vulnerable population, is now considered an important indicator of development. Health is increasingly being seen as a development issue rather than just a medical issue. Ill-health and poor access to health services are seen as indicators of poor economies and irresponsible health policies.

Health systems in contemporary societies are invariably dependent upon the political economy of the systems in which they operate. Polities in modern context and especially in the democratic set-ups can no longer ignore the health prescriptions suggested by WHO because such prescriptions also match to the felt needs and aspirations of politically conscious and numerically decisive citizens. But, the delivery systems do not always reflect the political idealism of 'health for all'. Economies, in the age of globalisation, look at health as the largest long-term investment for harnessing the human resources as well as marketing potentials. The inequalities created in political-economic systems did get reflected in terms of health opportunities and privileges.

The delivery of the health care system has to be determined by the health expectations of the people and these are also influenced by the social, cultural, economic and situational factors in the community. In a country characterised by inequalities of all sorts, seeking equilibrium between the health providers and health seekers is a great challenge. Social sciences are doing their best to create situations in which health facilities should not only be made available to the masses but also be made accessible for them.

Going by the socio-cultural and economic factors of health, studies reflect that poverty continues to be the greatest hurdle in ensuring good health in developing countries. Poor health drives the poor into absolute poverty, which in turn pushes them back into poor health status. Unavailability of food, malnutrition, poor sanitation, illiteracy, inadequate and ill-constructed housing, unemployment, poor working condition, etc., are other socio-cultural factors, which act as barriers in ensuring good health. Some other problems like food adulteration, unhygienic additives, food poisoning etc., also target the poor and the other marginalised communities specifically.

Despite the commitment to 'health for all', enormous health problems among Indian population and especially the vulnerable population suffering from spatio-stratal deprivations, continue to exist. While overall mortality has declined considerably, living standards of the masses are still among the poorest in the world. The major constraints facing the health sector are lack of resources, lack of an integrated support, poor involvement of NGOs, inadequate laboratory services, poor disease surveillance and response systems, and the heavy investments needed in dealing with communicable and non-communicable diseases. The problems of gender disparity still manifest themselves in various forms, as evidenced by the declining female to male population ratio, social stereotyping, violence at the domestic and social levels, and continuing open discrimination against the girl child, adolescent girls and women.

Further, in developing countries like India, health coverage continues to be an exception, rather than a rule. In India, less than 10 per cent of population currently has some form of health coverage. There is now enough evidence to indicate that the hardest hit by lack of health coverage are the poor, who have much higher levels of mortality, malnutrition and fertility than do the rich. A World Bank study based on the National Sample Survey 52nd round calculates that the poor-rich risk ratio is 2.5 for infant mortality, 2.8 for under-five mortality, 1.7 for childhood underweight and 2 for total fertility rate. The study further indicates that a higher percentage of the poor do not seek health care when ill: about 24 per cent of the poorest quintile does not seek care, compared to 9 per cent of the richest quintile (World Bank, 2001). The study reports that main reason for not seeking care is cost, especially for the poor.

Problems related to judicious distribution of health care facilities are many, such as, unequal access to health care services, limited attention to preventive methods, profit orientation of the agencies involved (especially private), malfunctioning and administrative weakness in government hospitals and health care centres, preponderance of unqualified and harmful health practitioners, discrimination against people with disabilities and high cost of medical care. The tribal communities of India, being the most marginalised in developmental context, are the largest victims of most of such maladies.

Studies also reveal that access to medical care is also positively associated with level of socio-economic development of the concerned communities. Facilities related to health care generally remain confined to developed areas. This reflects the spatial deprivations prevalent in health care accessibility. The tribal communities, who generally live in remote and less developed regions, are the greatest victims of this spatial deprivation.

The onslaught of new health hazards in the form of STDs/HIV/AIDS, which are sexually communicable complications, has added a newer dimension in the lives of entire humanity, transgressing the boundaries of east and west or developed and underdeveloped. Sexually transmitted diseases (STDs) are epidemics of tremendous health and economic consequences spread all over the world. Globally, more than 330 million new cases are being reported every year related to STDs. Of these, over 80 per cent are believed to occur in the developing countries. The total annual incidences of STDs in India are estimated to be around 5 per cent of the total population (NACO, 2000). In India, STDs have become one of the most prevalent communicable diseases, though very little data is available regarding their pattern.

The spread of STDs is closely related to social circumstances and human behaviour. People consider these diseases as something unmentionable and consequently hide them. These are often known as "*gupt rog*". The socio-cultural taboos related to sexuality are a barrier to STD prevention efforts on a number of levels. These efforts are also hampered by biological characteristics of STDs, societal problems, unbalanced mass media messages, lack of awareness, fragmentation of STD-related services, inadequate training of health care professionals and insufficient investment in STD prevention. Occurrence of HIV/AIDS, as an STD, has really made the world a difficult place to live in.

Tribal population in India are facing specific challenges of STDs because of variety of structural, socio-cultural and geographical reasons, such as illiteracy, poverty, non-availability of health care facilities etc. Further, unprotected sex, multiple partner relationship and commercial sex are other specific problems that make the tribal population more vulnerable to STDs. Very few studies have been conducted to detect the spread and magnitude of the problem keeping the tribal populace at the hub. Underreporting is itself a great problem among this unprivileged section of society. The dependence on quacks and local methods makes the situation very miserable as they often cause fatal casualties just because of ignorance.

The present work is an attempt to present the various issues related to health and diseases of Indian marginalised communities. India, a great country, has different patterns in its social structure. The health and disease conditions of its people are also varying. The level of interventions and the consequent changes are also not homogeneous. The dynamism of health in Indian communities is a pertinent issue, which attracts the attention of scholars as well as the common man towards it. The book is an effort to understand some aspects of the larger phenomenon.

The volume contains fifteen articles which are divided into three sections, namely, Conceptual and Constitutional Issues; Health, Disease and Social Structures; and Health Expenditure and Insurance. The papers reflect the views of various professionals and academicians related with health matters in different capacities. The focus of the book is to present a combination of theoretical frameworks and empirical realities. Orientations of individual authors may vary but the spirit of each of these articles is to explain and analyse how issues related to health are varying and how the ultimate sufferers of inherent discriminations in the world of health are the marginalised communities—be they the rural people, the tribal people or the persons living with STDs and HIV/AIDS.

Mohan Advani and Mohammad Akram look at the issues surrounding health and diseases in Indian context. This article is a ready reckoner for various concepts like health, public health, disease, health indicators (mortality, morbidity, average age etc.), health trends, health policies, health goals etc., and also pleads for increasing health coverage for common man and especially the unprivileged masses.

Mihir Desai quotes a good number of court judgments to explain how judiciary is playing a pivotal role in ensuring health for all. The state is committed to meet out the cost of health of its employees but the masses continue to be at the receiving end. Though the judiciary has been receptive and has recognised the right to health and health care as a fundamental right, globalisation and free markets pose a challenge which needs to be addressed by the courts, writes Desai.

For Sujata Krishnamurthi, health deprivation is becoming synonymous to class deprivation. The public health care in India is deficient. The main reasons are persistent under-funding, insufficient infrastructure including medicines and trained medical and para-medical staff, and inefficient functioning of district hospitals and sub-divisional centres. The dominating presence of the private players is changing the focus of health providers from care to profit. And, the ultimate looser are the poor masses.

The focus of the dominant bio-medical model of public health has always been on individual responsibility of self-care. Relegating to the background the larger socio-economic context in which lifestyles are 'created', public health policies have emphasised on behaviour modification. There is a tendency to focus on individual responsibility, which promotes a 'blaming culture'. The AIDS policy is one of the best examples of this reductionistic and myopic approach of public health. For an equitable and just society, a sound public health is vital. A meaningful discourse on public health of HIV/AIDS with transdisciplinary collaboration and universal sustainable improvement is yet looking for an alternative holistic vision. Using rigorous theoretical frameworks, Vijay Kumar Yadavendu analyses the philosophical background of the policy initiatives meant for combating spread of HIV/AIDS.

Tribal population constitutes about 8 per cent of India's population. Due to multi-dimensional factors, this population is facing many problems including ill-health, malnutrition and poor access to health care. B.V. Babu and Y.S. Kusuma take a holistic approach to understand the tribal health problems in India. The paper describes the situation of the both communicable and non-communicable diseases, as well as malnutrition, among Indian tribes. Also, it highlights the poor access and utilisation of health care services by this vulnerable population. The paper also talks about some social science perspectives during tackling the health and nutritional problems of the tribal population.

A person's attitudes, daily routine decisions regarding health maintenance, food habits and food serving practices are reflective of efforts on his or her part to maintain or restore himself or herself to his or her normal state. Madhu Nagla establishes how cultural structure of a particular society shows the pattern of health care. She deals with the study of attitudes and beliefs towards medicine and medical care systems in two different settings, i.e., urban and rural, in Haryana. She also analyses what sort of knowledge people have towards diseases and what they do to combat these. The results show how advice from science and health professionals tends to be filtered through existing beliefs and practices, and also through prevailing social relationships, thus minimising the impact.

B.L. Nagda writes in detail about the demographic realities of tribal population of Rajasthan. The data regarding tribal population in Rajasthan state have been collected through ethno- demographic literature, census, National Family Health

Survey (NFHS)-2 and other surveys conducted in the tribal areas of Rajasthan. He concludes that the number of health and medical institutions available, in tribal areas, is entirely inadequate to serve even minimum needs of the health.

Tribhu Nath Dubey and Supriya Seth advocate that the tribes of India are comparatively secluded, less educated, materially impoverished and underdeveloped groups and hence their health situation needs special attention. The wide gap between the health indicators of the rich and the poor is not only due to economic inequalities but also due to inequality of opportunities. For the authors, there is a need to think of a sub-plan for the vulnerable and deprived regions. Major thrust should be to help them reverse the situation through a well-planned, adequately financed community-oriented integrated health and development programmes with substantial participation from voluntary organisations.

Chakrapani Upadhayay, in his empirical study, explains that STDs are not just myth but a reality in the tribal world. Using statistical formulations, he assesses the level of awareness in relations to STDs, RTIs and STIs among the tribal population and develops correlation among the various factors involved. He also relates the problem with the cultural dogmas and the tribal way of life.

Mohammad Akram explains how prevalence and spread of STDs among the tribal population of Rajasthan is making life miserable for them. Making an extensive review of the behavioural aspects of tribal life, he has tried to develop some behaviour differentials, which are, somehow, responsible for the spread of STDs. The differentials can also be applied in other similar conditions and hence the findings are of great use in combating the menace.

Vani Verma, in her empirical study, delineates the socio-cultural aspects of persons suffering from STDs. Her findings reflect that education, marital status, migration, occupation, attitude and way of life play a significant role in spread of STDs and AIDS. Further, STDs also influence all these aspects of life and a vicious circle is developing which turns the problem into a gigantic one.

Despite the progress made in public health through improved hygiene and sanitary living conditions and development of germ theory of diseases through bacteriological researches, many tribal communities in India have deep faith in some magico-religious power involving forces beyond human comprehension for combating disease or ill-health. Balveer Singh delineates how the concept of health or illness gets institutionalised within the social and cultural milieus of every community and gets reflected through its level of development. For the Bhils of Rajasthan, it is their ethno-methodology, which provides motivational aspects related to the preventive or curative medical and health care. And, therefore, it also becomes obligatory for the health care system to come to the expectations of the people and serve their needs within their own psycho-social set-up.

N.K. Jha deals with the empirical, insightful and time-tested views of ancient Indian seer philosophers regarding the concept of sound health and ways and means to maintain it for the well-being of entire humanity. The whole gamut of Indian philosophy and oriental consciousness has emphasised the importance of celibacy or abstinence for the maintenance and sustenance of good health resulting in the procurement of hundred years of human age. He ventures upon analysing the views of Ayurvedācāryas and Yogacāryās in this regard and quotes extensively from the ancient texts to vindicate the assertions. Referring to the ancient texts, Jha concludes that STDs were not much prevalent in ancient India but maladies pertaining to sex did exist. The emphasis of the author has been on the obligatory adherence to moral values which can only be a deterrent to such a menace.

P.R. Sodani uses the data of a representative sample of households residing in tribal-sub plan (TSP) region of Rajasthan to investigate health seeking behaviour and household health care expenditure. Utilisation and expenditure for different types of providers are presented by rural/urban status. His findings indicate a high dependence on traditional practitioners in rural areas. In addition, rural households spend on health care one and a half times more than urban households. This study also reveals that rural people have a significantly higher burden of almost all components of indirect expenses for treatment. The results of this analysis are used to discuss the feasibility of implementing alternative health care financing reforms.

Health interventions can lead to economic growth and reduce inequity in developing countries. Given the rising expenditure on health care and state's as well as market's inability to protect the vulnerable section of the society, it becomes increasingly important to look at various alternatives of financing health care expenditure. Micro Health Insurance (MHI) is considered to be a potentially important source of financing health care expenditure and protecting the poor households from impoverishment. Gujarat state of India has a relatively large number of voluntary initiatives for providing health services in urban as well as rural areas. Akash Acharya analyses the NGO initiative of providing MHI to the poor of Gujarat. The paper by reviewing four NGO-run MHI schemes in Gujarat suggests that MHI schemes can devise a mechanism that enhances access to health care services, reduces the frequency of medical indebtedness and thus contributing positively to the health system goals.

The brief descriptions of the forthcoming chapters reinforce my initial postulate that deep-rooted health problems among Indian population and especially among the vulnerable population suffering from spatio-stratal deprivations continue to exist. Though the papers included in this volume cannot present the health deprivations existing among contemporary Indian societies in totality, the effort will be successful if it can present even a glimpse of that. The purpose of this book will be served if these papers can attain the attention of the policy makers, academicians, health professionals and all those who feel concerned towards the increasing discrimination inherent in the field of health and can help to mitigate them, no matter, how little!

I

Conceptual and Constitutional Issues

1

Health Concerns in India

Mohan Advani and Mohammad Akram

Health finds different interpretations from different perspectives. The biomedical approach which dominated the medical thought till the end of nineteenth century and based on the "germ theory of disease", views health as an "absence of diseases". This approach almost ignores the role of environmental, psychological and other socio-cultural factors in defining health. The ecological approach, views health as a dynamic equilibrium between man and his environment. For them, disease is maladjustment of the human organism to environment. The psychological approach states that health is not only related to body but also to mind and especially to the attitude of the individual. The socio-cultural approach considers health as a product of the social and community structure.

Health

Health is man's natural condition; health is his birthright. It is the result of living in accordance with natural laws pertaining to the body, mind and environment. These laws relate to fresh air, sunlight, diet, exercise, rest and relaxation, sleep, cleanliness, right attitude of mind, good habits and above all, lifestyle. The World Health Organisation (WHO) definition of health states that health is a state of complete physical, mental and social well-being, and not merely an absence of disease or infirmity. Health is multidimensional; three important dimensions of health are reflected in the WHO definition which are: physical, mental and social (Park, 2005: 13).

Physical Dimension

The state of physical health implies the notion of "perfect functioning" of the body. It conceptualises as a state in which every organ is in perfect harmony with the rest of body. The signs of physical health in an individual are – a good complexion, a clean skin, bright eyes, lustrous hair with a body well clothed with firm flesh, not too fat, a sweet breath, a good appetite, sound sleep, easy and coordinated movements.

Mental Dimension

Good mental health is the ability to respond to the many varied experiences of life with flexibility and a sense of purpose. The signs of a mentally healthy person are that he is free from internal conflicts, he is well adjusted and has a good self-control. Further, he is not overcome by emotions; he is not dominated by fear, anger, jealousy, guilt or worries; he faces problems and solves them intelligently.

Social Dimension

The social dimension of health includes the levels of social skills one possesses, social functioning and the ability to see oneself as a member of a large society. In general, social health takes into account that every individual is a part of a family and of wider community and focuses on social and economic conditions and well-being of the "whole person" in the context of his social network.

Holistic Approach to Health

The basic concept of holistic health is that a human being should be an integrated whole. Health professionals keep refining their definition of health to describe a state of total well-being. The constant interaction between all elements of the body makes it impossible to separate mental health from physical health, social well-being from spiritual well-being, or any one of these elements from the others. Each contributes to the status of the others. According to this total concept, better known as holistic concept, a healthy person is one who successfully experiences growth and development in all of these elements more or less at the same time.

Frazer Brockington identifies five stages in the preservation of health. The most important idea is the promotion of health by positive vital forces, that is by teaching physiological principles of healthy living or by providing good diet. The second stage seeks to prevent illness, chiefly by the application of medical knowledge in relation to a specific disease by inoculation, etc. The third, seeks to detect early departure from normal health with the object of bringing about a remedy, in advance for the established diseases. The fourth stage constitutes after care of sickness or injury in which remedies are sought for social factors and the last stage deals with the management of incurable sickness and it seeks for a worthwhile amelioration of it (Hobson, 1965).

Responsibility for Health

The health status of an individual, a community or a nation is determined by the interplay and integration of two ecological universes, the internal environment of the man himself and the external environment which surrounds him (Akram, 2005:

101). Health is on one hand a highly personal responsibility and on the other hand a major public concern. It involves the joint efforts of the whole social fabric, viz., the individual, the community and the state to protect and promote health (Park, 2005:20). The individual responsibility for health largely depends upon self-care which refers to those health-generating activities that are undertaken by the persons themselves. It comprises observance of simple rules of behaviour relating to diet, sleep, exercise, weight, hygiene, and the overall lifestyle. It also includes undertaking measures for preventing disease, treatment during illness and remaining aware about the biomedical and mental-psychological conditions of the individual concerned.

The individual and community responsibility are complementary and not antithetical to each other. The current trend is to "demedicalize" health and to involve the communities in a meaningful way. This implies a more active involvement of families and communities in health matters, viz., planning, implementation, utilisation, operation and evaluation of health services. The emphasis has shifted from health care for the people to health care by the people.

The responsibility for health does not end with the individual and community effort. In all civilised societies, the state assumes responsibility for health and welfare of its people. The Constitution of India, in the Directive Principles of State Policy asserts that health is a state responsibility. The Government of India has a health policy of its own and consistently designs a health policy to meet out the health requirements of its people.

Responsibility for health of the individuals is also shared by international agencies. The health of mankind requires the cooperation of governments, the people, national and international organisations both within and outside the United Nations system in achieving universal health goals.

Health System

Health system basically refers to the totality of formal efforts, commitments, personnel, institutions, economic resources, research efforts (both basic and applied) that a nation state or a society earmarks or devotes to illness, premature mortality, incapacitation, prevention, rehabilitation, and other health related problems. The word "system" is thus used in a fairly loose fashion and does not necessarily imply an organised and interrelated structure of activities, but it encompasses, all formal activities directed at health problems. The use of this expression thus parallels the view of society as a social system (Field, 1989: 10).

The goal of any medical or health care system is to organise for the provision and distribution of health services to those who need them, and to use the resources, knowledge, and technologies available to prevent and alleviate disease, disability, and suffering to the extent possible under prevailing conditions. There are alternative ways by which these goals may be pursued, and the form health institutions take is related to the form of other societal institutions and to the economic, organisational, and value context of the society of which they are a part. Further, there is no single ideal pattern of health organisation and each pattern of health care, that exists, involves both advantages and costs (Mechanic, 1978: 315-16).

Public Health

Health of an individual is important, no doubt, but when the collective health/community health, as a whole, as distinct from that of an individual, is taken into consideration, discussion centres round what is called public health. The Expert Committee of WHO has defined public health as the "science and art of preventing diseases, prolonging life and promoting mental and physical health and efficiency through organised community efforts for the sanitation of the environment, the control of communicable infection, the education of the individual's personal hygiene, the organisation of medical and nursing services for early diagnosis and preventive treatment of disease, the development of the social machinery to ensure to every individual a standard of living, adequate for the maintenance of health and so organising these benefits as to enable every citizen to realise his birth right of health and longevity" (WHO, 1952).

J.B. Grant, in a detailed and explanatory definition, states that public health is the science and art of social utilisation of scientific knowledge for medical protection by maintaining health, preventing disease, and curing disease through organised community efforts for (a) the hygiene of the environment, (b) the control of the community infections, (c) the education of the individual in principles of personal hygiene, (d) the organisation of medical and nursing service for the early diagnosis and preventive treatment of disease, and (e) the development of social machinery which will ensure to every individual in the community a standard of living adequate for the maintenance of health. As such, public health becomes social medicine and is primarily a field of social activity, applying practically every basic science directed towards a comprehensive programme of community service (Bagchi and Soman, 2005: 45).

The standard of health of people depends upon the levels of living, literacy and organisation of health services which in its turn depends on money, materials and institutions. Health is a logical prerequisite for socio-economic development as it affects both productivity and production. It is an important input for the development of man and thereby to social and economic development of the country. Achievement of good health and its maintenance is one of the universal values accepted by humanity as expressed through WHO's definition of health. This has changed the focus of the western medicine from treatment oriented, hospital based curative medicine to community based curative and preventive medicine. This shift has necessitated the knowledge about the community, its culture and ways of living.

Public health systems vary in different parts of the world, depending upon the prevalent health problems. In the developing world, where sanitation problems and limited medical resources persist, infectious diseases are the most significant threat to public health. Public health officials devote resources to establish sanitation systems and immunisation programmes to curb the spread of infectious diseases, and provide routine medical care to rural and isolated populations. In industrialised nations, sanitary food and water supplies and excellent medical resources have reduced rates of infectious disease. Instead, accidents and diseases such as lung cancer, heart attacks, and strokes are among the leading causes of death. In these areas, public health goals include education programmes to teach people how to prevent accidents and lessen their risk for disease, and the maintenance of the excellent disease prevention systems already established.

At the present time the field of public health is in a state of flux, for the concerns at every level of participation have changed enormously in recent years. The traditional concerns have receded in importance while new challenges in such fields as industrial health, nutrition, environmental pollution, accidents, health education and behaviour change, health-service research, social epidemiology and etiology and health care administration loom very large. The fast spread of AIDS and STDs has resulted in creation of new edifices to combat such epidemic-like maladies. The involvement of non-governmental organisations (NGOs) in health and especially public health issues are doing great jobs in creating awareness among the masses and ensuring community participation. The new studies conducted in the field of public health research and epidemiological research is giving ways to more realistic and pragmatic policy formulations.

Health Policies and Strategies

The health sector in India is characterised by: (i) a government sector that provides publicly financed and managed curative and preventive health services from primary to tertiary level, throughout the country and free of cost to the consumer (these account for about 18 per cent of the overall health spending and 0.9% of the GDP), and (ii) a fee-levying private sector that plays a dominant role in the provision of individual curative care through ambulatory services and accounts for about 82 per cent of the overall health expenditure and 4.2 per cent of the gross domestic product (GDP). Nationwide health care utilisation rates show that private health services are directed mainly at providing primary health care and financed from private resources, which could place a disproportionate burden on the poor. The provision of health care by the public sector is a responsibility shared by state, central and local governments, although it is effectively a state responsibility in terms of service delivery. State and local governments incur about three-quarters and the centre about one-quarter of public spending on health. The responsibility for health is at three levels. First, health is primarily a state responsibility. Second, the centre is responsible for health services in union territories without a legislature and is also responsible for developing and monitoring national standards and regulations, linking the states with funding agencies, and sponsoring numerous schemes for implementation by state governments. Third, both the centre and the states have a joint responsibility for programmes listed under the concurrent list. Goals and strategies for the public sector in health care are established through a consultative process involving all levels of government through the Central Council for Health and Family Welfare.

Financial Resources for Health

For the period 1998, the total health expenditure as a percentage of the GDP was 5.1 per cent. Public expenditure on health was 18 per cent of the total expenditure on health. The total government health expenditure as a percentage of the total government expenditure was 5.6 per cent.

Though India was committed to achieve 'Health for All' by the year 2000, the range and complexities of health issues have also been substantial. On the one hand the government has been struggling to combat communicable diseases while on the other having to cope with non-communicable diseases like diabetes, cancer, cardiovascular diseases, etc. In the constitutional provisions, health is primarily a state subject. States/union territories account for 76.26 per cent of the Eighth Plan health sector outlay as compared to 23.74 per cent from the centre. To augment the resources for health care, earmarked outlays are provided to state governments under the Minimum Needs Programme (MNP) with the explicit stipulation that these funds cannot be diverted elsewhere, and in case of diversion the central plan assistance to state governments will stand proportionately reduced. The family welfare/family-planning programme has been a 100 per cent centrally sponsored scheme from its inception. The financial outlay has also been increasing over the successive Five-Year Plan periods. In the 1996/97 budget, the allocation for health was increased by 21.6 per cent. Efforts have also been made to mobilise resources through various international organisations and UN agencies. The government has encouraged the involvement of private agencies in secondary and tertiary levels of health care.

Financial resources have been a major constraint to developing the primary and secondary levels of health care which are mainly provided by the government. Dependence, solely on government resources has been another constraint. For the future, the possibility of moving from strictly government-administered institutions to autonomous institutions or even to joint sector enterprises are options that are being discussed.

Physical Infrastructure

Since early 1990s, the emphasis has been towards consolidation and operationalisation, rather than on major expansion of the infrastructure. For this purpose, the following targets have been set:

1. One sub-centre staffed by a trained female health worker and a male health worker for a population of 5,000 in the plains and a population of 3,000 in hilly and tribal areas. As of 1998, 137,006 sub-centres had been established.
2. One primary health centre (PHC) staffed by a medical officer and other paramedical staff for a population of 30,000 in the plains and a population of 20,000 in hilly, tribal and backward areas. A PHC centre supervises six sub-centres. As of 1998, 23,179 PHCs had been established.
3. One community health centre (CHC) or an upgraded PHC with 30 beds and basic specialities covering a population of 80,000 to 120,000. The CHC acts as a referral centre for four PHCs. Up to 1998, 2,913 CHCs had been established.

Urban family welfare centres (FWCs) have been set up to provide family welfare/family planning services. In all, 1,529 urban FWCs are functioning (1996). The status of the infrastructure to deliver primary health care appears to be satisfactory but actual programme implementation needs a lot of improvement. Constraints include deficiency of skilled personnel, lack of basic facilities and simple equipment, etc. Also, staff shortages continue to plague the services at all levels. A substantial part of the physical infrastructure has still to be completed. A major factor has been that approved estimates/ norms for construction have not kept abreast with the rising estimates of actual construction costs. More than one quarter of the population now live in urban areas, with about 40-50 per cent of those in the metropolitan and large cities living in urban slums, with primary health care provided by health posts. Very often these health posts are outside slum areas, making access difficult. They also lack basic drugs, equipment and technical support. Consolidation, with attention to specific health needs of the community, will underpin future actions.

International Partnerships in Health

Various international organisations and UN agencies have continued to provide significant technical and material assistance which has had a positive impact. The various agencies include WHO, World Bank, UNICEF, UNFPA, USAID, Japanese Assistance, ODA (UK), SIDA, NORAD, DANIDA and German assistance. A National Institute of Biologicals has been set up as an autonomous organisation, with funding from the Government of India, the Japanese and USAID.

Health Policy in India

As per the WHO Country Health Profile – India (Trends in Policy Development), the main focus of the National Health Policy (NHP), adopted in 1983, was the formulation of an integrated and comprehensive approach towards future development of health services, appropriately supported by medical education and research, with special emphasis on PHC and related support services. During the Seventh Five-Year Plan, there was considerable achievement in terms of establishment of a health infrastructure, especially in rural areas. The Eighth Plan (1992-97) identified "human development" as its main focus, with health and population control listed as two of the six priority objectives. It was emphasised that health facilities must reach the entire population by the end of the Eighth Plan. The Plan also identified people's initiative and participation as a key element. With the enactment of the 73rd Constitutional Amendment Act (1992), Panchayati Raj Institutions (PRIs) were revitalised and a process of democratic decentralisation ushered in, with similar provisions made for urban local bodies, municipalities and Nagar Palikas.

Recognising the importance of sustainable development, a national conservation strategy and a policy statement on environment and development were formulated in 1992 to bring environmental considerations into the developmental process. Linkages were drawn between poverty, population growth and the environment. The NHP identified nutrition as a problem needing urgent attention and in 1993 a National Nutrition Policy was formulated with long- and short-term strategies.

The vertically structured family welfare programme needed to be replaced by a more democratic, decentralised alternative. In 1994 a draft national population policy was submitted to parliament as well as a revised report in 1996. It advocated a holistic, multisectoral approach towards population stabilisation, with no targets for specific contraceptive methods except for achieving a national average total fertility rate (TFR) of 2.1 by the year 2010. This has resulted in a radical shift in implementation from centrally fixed targets to a target-free dispensation through a decentralised, participatory approach. A Population and Social Development Commission was also established in support of the population policy.

India has accepted the recommendations of the International Conference on Population and Development (ICPD) (1994) and has also ratified various international conventions for securing equal rights for women. Following the World Summit on Survival, Protection and Development of Children in 1990, India formulated a Plan of Action for Children in 1992 with actions that directly and indirectly affect child health.

Despite the commitment to 'Health for All', enormous health problems still need to be addressed. While overall mortality has declined considerably, living standards are still among the poorest in the world. The major constraints facing the health sector are lack of resources, lack of an integrated support, poor involvement of NGOs, inadequate laboratory services, poor disease surveillance and response systems, and the heavy investments needed in dealing with non-communicable diseases. The problems of gender disparity still manifest themselves in various forms, as evidenced by the declining female to male population ratio, social stereotyping, violence at the domestic and social level, and continuing open discrimination against the girl child, adolescent girls and women.

Thus, the period after the last National Health Plan was announced in 1983, has seen major developments in India. There has been an increase in mortality through 'lifestyle diseases' – diabetes, cancer and cardiovascular diseases. The increase in life expectancy has increased the requirement for geriatric care. Similarly, the increasing burden of trauma cases is also a significant public health problem. The changed circumstances relating to the health sector of the country since 1983 have generated a situation in which the government has undertaken steps to formulate a new policy framework as the National Health Policy, 2001.

The NHP, 2001 attempts to set out a new policy framework for the accelerated achievement of public health goals in the socio-economic circumstances currently prevailing in the country.

Trends in Health Status in India

Life expectancy

It refers to average expected life of an individual at the time of his birth. When expected average life of an individual is long, it reflects good state of health and control over morbidity conditions. It is estimated for both sexes separately. For the period 1996-2001, the life expectancy at birth is estimated to be 62.36 years for males and 63.39 years for females. In 1991, the sex ratio was 927 females per 1,000 males which increased to 933 in 2001. To ensure the continued improvement in life expectancy, the health care delivery infrastructure is being expanded, Maternal and Child Health (MCH) care is being improved, specific programmes such as the expanded programme on immunisation (EPI), introduction of oral rehydration therapy (ORT), etc., are being strengthened, and efforts are continuing to contain locally endemic diseases.

Mortality

It generally refers to death or end of life. Infant mortality rate (IMR) is the ratio of deaths under one year of age in a given year to the total number of live births in the same year; usually expressed as a rate per 1,000 live births. It was reported to be 68 per 1,000 live births in 1994-98 and the maternal mortality ratio (MMR) for 1998 was estimated at 407 per 100,000 live births. Estimates for 1996 of the number of deaths per year in children under five years from diarrhoeal diseases was 840,000, from acute respiratory infections 600,000 and from measles 330,000. Deaths from malaria were reported to be 1,061 (1995) and 1,057 (1999), cardiovascular diseases 2,386,000 (1990), traffic accidents 45,670 (1993), and work accidents 543 (1993). Between 1986 and 1999 the crude death rate (CDR) declined from 11.1 to 8.7 per 1,000 population. Between 1980 and 1998 the IMR declined from 114 to 68, the leading causes of death being diseases of circulatory system, infections and parasitic diseases, injury, poisoning, perinatal conditions, and diseases of respiratory system. The number of reported accidental deaths in 1993 was 11,125 and 80,000 in 1998. The main constraints are low literacy and income levels, socio-cultural beliefs and practices, and sub-optimal utilisation of health facilities.

Morbidity

Mortality rate alone is not a good indicator of state of health of a society because death, after certain age is also natural. Mortality rate does not reveal the burden of ill-health in a community. Morbidity, on the other hand, reflects the number of persons affected with some disease and hence indicates ill-health. The number of reported cases of the following diseases were: leprosy 560,000 (2000), malaria 2,276,788 (1999), measles 26,986 (1991), neonatal tetanus 1,896 (1995), polio 142 (2000/2001), and tuberculosis 1,223,127 (1999). The vaccine-preventable diseases have declined significantly since implementation of the EPI. In India about 14 million people are estimated to be suffering from active tuberculosis and about 0.5 million die of the disease each year. Currently, short-term chemotherapy using Directly Observed Treatment Short Course (DOTS) has been introduced and accessibility to tuberculosis treatment centres improved. The prevalence of leprosy has declined from about 39 per 10,000 population in 1985 to about 7 per 10,000 in 1995 and further down to 3.7 in 2000. The spectacular reduction in this disease has been due to the new regimen of multi-drug therapy. The number of new cases detected annually has, however, remained more or less the same, at about 0.5 million.

Disability

Disability prevalence rates per 100,000 population estimated in 1994 are as follows: physical disability 3,574, visual disability 827, hearing 806, speech 510, and locomotor disability 2,041. The incidence rates per 100,000 population of these disabilities are: physical 173, visual 45, hearing 27, speech 10 and locomotor disability 105.

The main cause of blindness is cataract (80.1%), with about 6.5 million (2000) persons blind due to cataract. The national blindness control programme is centrally sponsored with a four-pronged strategy to strengthen service delivery, develop human resources, promote outreach activities and develop institutional capacity.

Due to changing lifestyles, mental disorders are likely to increase in the future. The total number of mental disorders treated in specialised mental hospitals was 48,396 in 1991 and 38,323 in 1992. The majority of cases have been diagnosed as suffering from psychosis (85.7%) (WHO Country Health Profile – India).

Health Insurance

Health care promotion has been an integral component of all national health and family welfare programmes. Health status of a population and especially of the vulnerable population is now considered an important indicator of development. Health is increasingly being seen as a development issue rather than just a medical issue. Ill-health and poor access to health services are being seen as indicator of poor economies and irresponsible health policies.

In developing countries like India, health coverage continues to be an exception, rather than a rule. In India, less than 10 per cent of population currently has some form of health coverage. There is now enough evidence to indicate that the hardest hit by lack of health coverage are the poor, who have much higher levels of mortality, malnutrition and fertility than do the rich (Gupta and Trivedi, 2005: 4132). A World Bank study based on the National Sample Survey 52nd round calculates that the poor-rich risk ratio is 2.5 for infant mortality, 2.8 for under-five mortality, 1.7 for childhood underweight and 2 for total fertility rate. The study also indicates that a higher percentage of the poor do not seek health care when ill: about 24 per cent of the poorest quintile does not seek care, compared to 9 per cent of the richest quintile (World Bank, 2001). The study reports that main reason for not seeking care is cost, especially for the poor.

For the period 1998, the total health expenditure as a percentage of the GDP was 5.1 per cent. Public expenditure on health was 18 per cent of the total expenditure on health and the rest is shared by the private sector. The total government health expenditure as a percentage of the total government expenditure was 5.6 per cent. Private sector in India accounts for more than 80 per cent of all health spending, one of the highest proportions of private spending found anywhere in the world (World Bank, 2002). Given the rising expenditure on health care and the inability of the state and the market to protect the vulnerable sections of society, it becomes increasingly important to look at various alternatives for financing this expenditure (Acharya and Ranson, 2005: 4143).

Thus, there is an urgent need to provide access to affordable health care in a sustainable manner. This could be based on an underlying strategy of preventive rather than curative medical care. One viable proposition is an insurance model that will support millions across India's rural hinterland through a network of hospitals. Roughly translated it means, "Insuring Affordable Health Care". The Yashaswini Health Insurance Scheme introduced in Karnataka in 2003 is a glaring example of this in which members of various cooperatives receive an insurance cover against an extensive list of surgical procedures for a nominal premium of Rs 60 per annum. Another private initiative, Arogya Raksha Yojna is a comprehensive health insurance scheme that goes beyond surgeries and encompasses hospitalisation, free medical consultations and low-cost medicines for a premium of Rs 120 per annum. Both these programmes rely on a network of government hospitals (in the case of the Yashaswani programme) and private hospitals and clinics (in the Arogya Raksha model), to provide quality health care (Shaw, 2005).

The recent proposition by the Insurance Regulatory and Development Authority (IRDA) to allow insurance companies to issue composite micro-insurance policies is also a step forward in the desired direction. Under this scheme, an assured sum of anywhere between Rs 5,000 and Rs 50,000 will cover life, health, household, fire and motor accident risks. However, the modalities for the composite insurance are yet to be decided. India has been grappling with the objective of 'Health for All' for a while now, wondering how exactly to meet this. It is time to understand that Health for All can happen if we adopt a model of 'Health Coverage for All' (Gupta and Trivedi, 2005: 4137).

Millennium Development Goals (MDGs): Targets and Indicators Related to Health

Health and the MDGs

In September 2000, the largest-ever gathering of Heads of State ushered in the new millennium by adopting the UN Millennium Declaration. The Declaration, endorsed by 189 countries, was then translated into a roadmap setting out goals to be reached by 2015.

The eight MDGs build on agreements made at United Nations conferences in the 1990s and represent commitments to reduce poverty and hunger, and to tackle ill-health, gender inequality, lack of education, lack of access to clean water and environmental degradation (Table 1.1). The MDGs are framed as a compact, which recognises the contribution that developed countries can make through trade, development assistance, debt relief, access to essential medicines and technology transfer.

Three out of eight goals, eight of the 16 targets and 18 of the 48 indicators relate directly to health. Health is also an

Table 1.1

Goals, Targets and Indicators Related to Health

Goals		*Targets*		*Indicators*
Goal 1	Eradicate extreme poverty and hunger	1.	Half between 1990 and 2015, the proportion of people whose income is less than one dollar a day	
		2.	Half between 1990 and 2015, the proportion of people who suffer from hunger	Prevalence of underweight children under five years of age, proportion of population below minimum level of dietary energy consumption
Goal 2:	Achieve universal primary education	3.	Ensure that, by 2015, children everywhere, boys and girls alike, will be able to complete a full course of primary schooling	
Goal 3:	Promote gender equality and empower women	4.	Eliminate gender disparity in primary and secondary education, preferably by 2005, and at all levels of education no later than 2015	
Goal 4:	Reduce child mortality	5.	Reduce by two-thirds, between 1990 and 2015, the under-five mortality rate	Under-five mortality rate infant mortality rate, proportion of one-year-old children immunised against measles
Goal 5:	Improve maternal health	6.	Reduce by three-quarters, between 1990 and 2015, the maternal mortality ratio	Maternal mortality ratio, proportion of births attended by skilled health personnel

Contd...

Contd...

Goal 6:	Combat HIV/AIDS, Malaria and other diseases	7.	Have halted by 2015 and begun to reverse the spread of HIV/AIDS	HIV prevalence among pregnant women aged 15-24 years. Condom use rate of the contraceptive prevalence rate. Ratio of school attendance of orphans to school attendance of non-orphans aged 10-14 years
		8.	Have halted by 2015 and begun to reverse the incidence of malaria and other major diseases	Prevalence and death rates associated with malaria. Proportion of population in malaria-risk areas using effective malaria prevention and treatment measures. Prevalence and death rates associated with tuberculosis. Proportion of tuberculosis cases detected and cured under DOTS (Directly Observed Treatment Short-course)
Goal 7:	Ensure environmental sustainability	9.	Integrate the principles of sustainable development into country policies and programmes and reverse the loss of environmental resources	Proportion of population using solid fuels
		10	Half by 2015 the proportion of people without sustainable access to safe drinking-water and sanitation	Proportion of population with sustainable access to an improved water source, urban and rural
		11.	By 2020 to have achieved a significant improvement in the lives of at least 100 million slum dwellers	Proportion of population with access to improved sanitation, urban and rural
Goal 8:	Develop a global partnership for development	12.	Develop further an open, rule-based, predictable, non-discriminatory trading and financial system	

Contd...

Contd...

	13. Address the special needs of the least developed countries	
	14. Address the special needs of landlocked countries and small island developing states	
	15. Deal comprehensively with the debt problems of developing countries through national and international measures in order to make debt sustainable in the long term	
	16. In cooperation with developing countries, develop and implement strategies for decent and productive work for youth	
	17. In cooperation with pharmaceutical companies, provide access to affordable, essential drugs in developing countries	Proportion of population with access to affordable essential drugs on a sustainable basis
	18. In cooperation with the private sector, make available the benefits of new technologies, especially information and communications	

important contributor to several other goals. The significance of the MDGs lies in the linkages between them: they are a mutually reinforcing framework to improve overall human development. The MDGs provide a vision of development in which health and education are squarely at the centre. Since their adoption, no one has been able to say that development is just about economic growth.

The MDGs do not say everything that needs to be said about health and development. They say nothing about the importance of effective health systems which are essential to the achievement of all health goals, about reproductive health or non-communicable diseases. We therefore have to understand the MDGs as a form of shorthand for some of the most important outcomes that development should achieve:

- fewer women dying in childbirth;
- more children surviving the early years of life;
- dealing with the catastrophe of HIV/AIDS;
- making sure people have access to life-saving drugs; and
- better health – in all its forms – making a major contribution to the reduction of poverty.

Health status of a nation is difficult to define only in terms of some identified indicators. Health of a nation or community is a product of many factors and forces that combine and interact with each other. Some important factors that we have discussed earlier, like life expectancy, infant mortality and maternal mortality rates, birth rate, nutrition level, etc., give some idea about the prevalent health scenario in a nation. Besides, economic growth, per capita income, employment, education, literacy, health awareness, hygiene conditions, sanitation, birth control measures, availability of safe drinking water, access to health care centre, health insurance and government's commitment for equitable growth are other factors that determine the health status of the nation.

The health condition of Indian population has improved significantly over the past five decades. Life expectancy has risen from 33 years to 64 years. The infant mortality rate has fallen from 148 to 64 per thousand. The crude birth rate has declined from 41 to 25 and the crude death rate has fallen from 25 to 8.1. The couple protection rate and total fertility rate have also improved substantially. One of the main reasons for such significant change in health condition is the fact that India is the first country in the world to launch a family planning programme, way back, in 1951. Since then, hundreds of programmes have been launched to control all possible dimensions of health and disease.

However, the goal of health for all, is still not attained. The government has introduced the National Rural Health Mission (NRHM) recently to fulfil the unfulfilled agenda. It has introduced several new variables to ensure health for all and public-private partnership is the new strategy. But, increasing cost of health is a great challenge. The government still needs new mechanism to meet out the cost of health for the poor. A proper coordination between health, hygiene, population and political economy is still lacking. The government needs to make health facilities not only available, but also accessible. Let us hope for a bright future.

References

Acharya, A., and Ranson, M.K., 2005, "Health Care Financing for the Poor: Community-based Health Insurance Schemes in Gujarat", *Economic and Political Weekly*, Vol. XL, No. 38, pp. 4141-4150, September 17-23.

Akram, M., 2005, "Sustainable Development, Health and STDs: A Study of Tribal Society of Rajasthan", *Social Change*, Vol. 35, No. 3, September, pp. 99-110.

Bagchi, A.K., and Soman, K., 2005, *Maladies, Preventives and Curatives, Debates in Public Health in India*, New Delhi: Tulika Books.

Field, M.G., 1989, *Success and Crisis in National Health Systems: A Comparative Approach*, New York: Routledge.

Gupta, I., and Trivedi, M., 2005, "Social Health Insurance Redefined: Health For All through Coverage for All", *Economic and Political Weekly*, Vol. XL, No. 38, pp. 4132-4140, September 17-23.

Hobson, W. (ed.), 1965, *The Theory and Practice of Public Health*, New York, p. 344.

Mechanic, David, 1978, *Medical Sociology*, New York: The Free Press, pp. 315-16.

Park, K., 2005, *Park's Text Book of Preventive and Social Medicine*, Jabalpur: Banarsidas Bhanot Publishers.

Shaw, K.M., 2005, *Times of India*, Delhi Edition, October 23.

WHO, 1952, *Report of Expert Committee on Public Health Administration.*

WHO, 1976, *Health Aspects of Human Rights*, Geneva.

WHO, *Country Health Profile – India (Trends in Policy Development)* http://w3.whosea.org/en/Section313/Section1519.htm

World Bank, 2001, India-Raising the Sites: Better Health Systems for India's Poor. Quoted in Gupta and Trivedi, 2005.

World Bank, 2002, "India: Raising the Sites–Better Health Systems for India's Poor: Findings, Analysis and Options", Health, Nutrition and Population Series, Washington, D.C. Qouted in Acharya and Ranson, 2005.

http://encyclopedia.thefreedictionary.com

Microsoft Encarta Encyclopedia Deluxe (2004).

2

Judicial Response to Health Care

Mihir Desai

Until the early 1980s judicial response to health-related issues in India was essentially centred around cases of medical negligence. Even these cases were few and far between. There were two developments in the 1980s, which led to a marked increase in health-related litigation. First was the establishment of consumer courts that made it cheaper and speedier to sue doctors for medical negligence. Second, the growth of public interest litigation and one of its offshoots being recognition of health and health care as a fundamental right.

This paper deals mainly with two themes: (1) fundamental right to health, and (2) emergency health care.

Right to Health as a Fundamental Right

Article 21 of the Indian Constitution says, "No person shall be deprived of his life or personal liberty except through procedure established by law".

Reprinted (with some modifications) with permission from *Combat Law*, Vol. 4, Issue 4 (Novemer-December, 2005) and duly acknowledged.

Till the 1970s by and large the courts had interpreted "life" literally, i.e., right to exist. It was in late 1970s onwards that an expanded meaning started to be given to the word "life". Over the years it has come to be accepted that life does not only mean animal existence but the life of a dignified human being with all its concomitant attributes. This would include a healthy environment and effective health care facilities.

To begin with, the right to health as a fundamental right grew as an offshoot of the environmental litigation. Pollution-free environment as a fundamental right presupposes right to health as a fundamental right. Logically, the explicit recognition of the fundamental right to health should have preceded the fundamental right to good environment. However, the development of jurisprudence in this branch has been reverse. To begin with, right to decent environment was recognised and from that followed the right to public health, health and health care. Even while dealing directly with right to health, the first issue concerns employees' health.

Employees' Right to Health

In 1991, in *C.E.S.C. Ltd. v. Subhas Chandra*, the Supreme Court placed reliance on international instruments and declared that right to health is a fundamental right. It went further and observed that health is not merely absence of sickness and observed:

> 33. ...In the light of Arts. 22 to 25 of the Universal Declaration of Human Rights, International Convention on Economic, Social and Cultural Rights, and in the light of socio-economic justice assured in our Constitution, right to health is a fundamental human right to workmen. The maintenance of health is a most imperative constitutional goal

> whose realization requires interaction by many social and economic factors.

In *CERC v. Union of India*, the Supreme Court was dealing with the rights of workers in asbestos manufacturing and health hazards related to it. It observed:

> 27. Therefore, we hold that right to health, medical aid to protect the health and vigour of a worker while in service or post retirement is a fundamental right under Article 21, read with Articles 39(e), 41, 43, 48A and all related to Articles and fundamental human rights to make the life of the workman meaningful and purposeful with dignity of person.

Similarly, in *State of Punjab v. Mohinder Singh Chawla,* dealing with rights of government employees to health care, the Supreme Court observed:

> It is now settled law that right to health is an integral to right to life. Government has constitutional obligation to provide the health facilities. If the Government servant has suffered an ailment, which requires treatment at a specialized, approved hospital and on reference whereat the Government servant had undergone such treatment therein, it is but the duty of the State to bear the expenditure incurred by the Government servant. Expenditure, thus, incurred requires to be reimbursed by the State to the employee.

Is it only State Responsibility?

In *Virender Gaur v. State of Haryana*, 1995 (2) SCC 577, the Supreme Court held that environmental, ecological, air and water pollution, etc., should be regarded as amounting to violation of right to health guaranteed by Article 21 of the Constitution. In *Kirloskar Brothers Ltd. v. Employees' State Insurance Corporation*, the Supreme Court held that right to health and medical care is a fundamental right under Article 21 read with Articles 39(e), 41 and 43. It is also relevant to notice as per the judgment of the Supreme Court in *Vincent Panikurlangara v. Union of India*, AIR 1987 SC 990-(1987)2 SCC165, "In a welfare state, therefore, it is the obligation of the State to ensure the creation and the sustaining of conditions congenial to good health".

But having recognised that right to health and health care is a fundamental right what follows? Fundamental rights are generally available only against the state. They prescribe the obligations of the state. In a poverty-ridden country like India, does it mean that the state must provide free medical health care facilities to all? In a situation where there is increasing privatisation of health care systems, where the annual budget for health is reducing, where the cost of health education is growing exponentially this seems very unlikely. No court has yet said that the state is bound to provide free medical care to all citizens.

Quality of Health Care

The other aspect would of course be the quality of health care provided by the state. Infrastructure in not just primary health care centres but even in government-run hospitals in metropolitan cities is crumbling. These institutions are plagued by lack of enough beds, sufficient medicines and other similar problems. The courts including the Supreme Court have not adequately dealt with this aspect. They have mainly been concerned with pious declarations of health being a fundamental right and peripheral and not so peripheral issues such as rights of government employees to be treated in government hospitals, emergency medical care and the like. But in a case dealing with bad infrastructure in public hospitals the Allahabad High Court held:

> It is indeed true that most of the Government Hospitals in Allahabad are in a very bad shape and need drastic improvement so that the Public is given proper medical treatment. Anyone who goes to the Government Hospitals in Allahabad will find distressing sanitary and hygienic conditions. The poor people, particularly, are not properly looked after and not given proper medical treatment. Consequently, most people who can afford it go to private nursing homes or private clinics. ...All this needs to be thoroughly investigated. This is a welfare State, and the people have a right to get proper medical treatment. In this connection, it may be mentioned that in U.S.A. and Canada there is a law that no hospital can refuse medical treatment of a person on the ground of his poverty or inability to pay. In our opinion Article 21 of the Constitution, as interpreted in a series of judgments of the Supreme Court, has the same legal effect.

Statutory Duties

In the case of *B. Poonam Sharma v. Union of India*, the police took the petitioner's husband who had met with an accident into custody as they suspected him of drunken driving. The deceased had suffered one inch cut on his head and he was taken to a government hospital for first aid. The government doctor stitched up the wound and prescribed ibuprofen tablets. Thereafter, police charged him under the Motor Vehicles Act and put him behind bars. At night, the deceased complained of severe headache and he was taken back to the same doctor who gave the deceased some more ibuprofen tablets and sent him back without examining him. Next day he was released on bail. When the condition of the deceased deteriorated, his relatives took him back to the same hospital. The hospital took X-Rays and CAT scan that showed brain haemorrhage, and he was immediately referred to a specialist hospital but succumbed to his injuries at the time of admission. Petitioner invoked writ jurisdiction of High Court under Article 226 and sought relief against the alleged negligence on part of the government doctor and police that caused the death of the petitioner's husband.

The High Court held that the instant case was not of an error of judgment as within a few hours patient was brought back complaining of severe headache yet no further treatment was given. The court held that every doctor at the government hospital having regard to the paramount importance of preservation of human life is under statutory obligation to extend his services with due expertise. Hence, respondent was directed to pay Rs 2 lakh as compensation under public law for violation of fundamental rights of petitioner's husband.

In *Marri Yadamma v. State of Andhra Pradesh*, the deceased was an under-trial who died of 'congestive cardiac failure'. The petition was filed by his spouse alleging negligence on part of the jail authorities and jail doctor in not providing appropriate treatment on time or referring to a specialist to determine the root cause of the ailment. The High Court in this case observed that the condition of the deceased at the time of his death was such that could have developed over a period of time and not immediately. Thus, it was abundantly clear that no care or caution was taken by the respondents to get the deceased examined by a surgeon or a specialist, even though he was complaining of ailments very often. The court stated that on arrest a prisoner merely loses his right to free movement. His all other rights including right to medical treatment remains intact and it cannot be violated. The jail authorities had infringed fundamental right of the deceased, therefore the State was liable to compensate his widow as a public law remedy for an amount of Rs 2 lakh.

Mental Health and Courts

In the case of death of 25 chained inmates in an asylum fire in Tamil Nadu, in *Re. v. Union of India*, the petitioners sought directions for implementation of provisions of Mental Health

Act, 1987 to prevent another mishap of the kind in mental asylum in Tamil Nadu.

In light of the provisions of Mental Health Act, Supreme Court issued following directions for its implementation:

(i) Every state and union territory must undertake a district-wise survey of all registered/unregistered bodies, by whatever name called, purporting to offer psychiatric/mental health care. All such bodies should be granted or refused licence depending upon whether minimum prescribed standards are fulfilled or not. In case licence is rejected, it shall be the responsibility of SHO of the concerned police station to ensure that the body stops functioning and patients are shifted to governmental mental hospitals.

(ii) Chief Secretary or Additional Chief Secretary designated by him shall be the nodal agency to coordinate all activities involved in implementation of the Mental Health Act, 1987, the Persons with Disabilities (Equal Opportunities, Protection of Rights and Full Participation) Act, 1995 and National Trust for Welfare of Persons with Autism, Cerebral Palsy, Mental Retardation, and Multiple Disability Act, 1999. He shall ensure that there are no jurisdictional problems or impediments to the effective implementation of the three Acts between different Ministries or Departments. At the central level, Cabinet Secretary, Government of India or any Secretary designated by him shall be the nodal agency for the same purpose.

Emergency Health Care

One of the major issues concerning health care has been the obligation of doctors to provide emergency health care. In the case of *Paschim Banga Khet Mazdoor Samity v. State of West Bengal* the Supreme Court observed that providing adequate medical facilities is an essential part of the obligation undertaken by the state in a welfare state. And, the failure on the part of a government hospital to provide timely medical treatment to a person in need of such treatment results in violation of his right to life guaranteed under Article 21.

The issue before Supreme Court was the legal obligation of government to provide facilities in government hospitals for treatment of persons who had sustained serious injuries and required immediate medical attention. In the case before the court, petitioner who had suffered brain haemorrhage in a fall from the train was denied treatment at various government hospitals because of non-availability of beds. Government justified its action on the ground that the petitioner could not have been kept on floor of a hospital or trolley because such arrangement of treatment was fraught with grave risks of cross-infection and lack of facility for proper post-operative care. It further argued that state hospitals cater to the need of poor and indigent patients as of the total number of beds maintained by the state government all over the state, 90 per cent are free beds for treatment of such patients.

During the pendency of the case, the state government appointed an enquiry committee to investigate the matter. The state government adopted various recommendations made by the enquiry committee. Apart from the recommendations of the enquiry committee, the Supreme Court made certain additional directions in respect of serious medical cases:

1. Adequate facilities be provided at the Primary Health Centres where the patient can be given basic treatment and his condition stabilised.
2. At the district and sub-divisional level it should be upgraded so that serious cases can be treated there.
3. Facilities for giving specialist treatment should be increased and having regard to the growing need, it must be made available at the district and sub-divisional level hospitals.

4. In order to ensure availability of bed in an emergency at state level hospitals, there should be a centralised communication system so that the patient can be sent immediately to the hospital where bed is available in respect of the treatment, which is required.
5. Proper arrangement of ambulance should be made for transport of a patient from the primary health centre to the district hospital or sub-divisional hospital to the state hospital.
6. Ambulance should be adequately provided with necessary equipment and medical personnel.

The Supreme Court observed that though for implementation of the above directions financial resources would be required, but at the same time it cannot be ignored that it is the constitutional obligation of state to provide adequate medical services to the people. The apex court also observed: "In the context of the constitutional obligation to provide free legal aid to a poor accused this Court has held that the State cannot avoid its constitutional obligation in that regard on account of financial constraints (*Khatri II v. State of Bihar*). These observations will apply with equal, if not greater, force in the matter of discharge of constitutional obligation of the state to provide medical aid to preserve human life. In the matter of allocation of funds for medical services the said constitutional obligation of the State has to be kept in view." The Supreme Court held that it was necessary that a time-bound plan for providing these services should be chalked out keeping the above in mind.

This case arose out of an incident in West Bengal. Other states were not parties to the case. Also, the enquiry committee was concerned with West Bengal and the directions were also given by the West Bengal government. The Supreme Court, however, observed that other states, though not parties, should also take necessary steps as set out in the judgment. Thus, all the directions referred to above, would be equally applicable to other states in the country.

It is to be noted that though the responsibility of the state and government hospitals is well provided by a radical interpretation of the Constitution, there is no definite corresponding legal duty imposed on private hospitals and practitioners to treat emergency cases. The above judgments focus on the duty of state and government hospitals.

Medico-legal Cases

Parmanand Katara v. Union of India was filed by a human right activist seeking directions against Union of India that every injured citizen brought for treatment should be instantaneously given medical aid to preserve life and thereafter the procedural criminal law should be allowed. It was widely observed that when accident victims or victims of crimes are brought to hospitals; doctors refuse to touch them till the police formalities are completed. Some doctors do not treat them even after this for fear of having to attend courts. The Supreme Court held:

> There is no legal impediment for a medical professional when he is called upon or requested to attend to an injured person needing his medical assistance immediately. The effort to save the person should be the top priority not only of the medical professional but even of the police or any other citizen who happens to be connected with the matter or happens to notice an incident or a situation. Every doctor whether at a Government hospital or otherwise has the professional obligation to extend his services with due expertise for protecting life. No law or State action can intervene to avoid delay the discharge of the paramount obligation case upon the members of the medical profession. The obligation being total, absolute and paramount, laws of procedure whether in statutes or otherwise which would interfere with discharge of

this obligation cannot be sustained and must, therefore, give way..."

The Supreme Court and the High Courts have been intervening in a much more active manner in the last few years on the issue of health and health care. But again, unless they start looking into the impact of patents and drug price control as also the obligations of private hospitals, the effect is bound to be limited.

(*Acknowledgement*: The author is indebted to Deepti Chand for the research done by her, which has been the basis of portions of this article.)

3

Right to Life

A Prerogative of the Wealthy?

Sujata Krishnamurthi

The current direction of India's health care policy is in the same trajectory as that of Argentina. The United Nations Development Programme's (UNDP) Human Development Report (HDR) indicates India's public spending on health is among the lowest in the world – just 4 US $ a person a year or 0.9 per cent of its gross domestic product (GDP). Of the 175 countries documented by the HDR, only four have a lower public spending on health than India. In sharp contrast, India ranks an impressive 18th in private health care spending (4.2% of GDP). Such a harsh distinction exists only for very few countries.

India's health care system, comprising government and private sectors, barely covers half its population. This public sector health infrastructure has about five lakh doctors, 7.4 lakh nurses, 3.5 lakh chemists, 15,000 hospitals and 8,70,000 beds. It is a three-tier structure comprising some 23,000 primary health centres (PHCs), 1,37,000 sub-centres and 3,000

Reprinted with permission from *Combat Law*, Vol. 4, Issue 4 (November-December, 2005) and duly acknowledged.

community health centres (CHCs), serving the semi-urban and rural areas.

The Bhore Committee (1964) report stated that comprehensive health care should be accessible to everyone, irrespective of the ability to pay. In its 1983 National Health Policy (NHP), the government had declared a goal, "health for all by the year 2000". By the end of the 1980s, however, it began to openly accept its inability to achieve health goals and began to accord a prominent role to the private sector in the delivery of health care. With the advent of structural adjustment policies in 1990s, inequalities in access to health care widened. The stagnation of budgetary allocation for health care, sky rocketing drug prices and an unregulated privatisation have sounded the death knell for universal access to health care.

The World Trade Organisation (WTO), through the General Agreement on Trade In Services (GATS), is creating potential extra pressure for the privatisation of public services, especially health care. The key element in GATS is for countries to make "commitments" to open a sector to trade. Health services are also included under the GATS heading of "professional services", which covers medical and dental services as well as the category of "services provided by midwives, nurses, physiotherapists and paramedical personnel".

The key factors on the ground are the multinational and trans-national corporations, including pharmaceutical, insurance and health care companies, which are in the forefront of pushing health services as a tradable commodity.

The commitment of India under the Trade-Related Aspects of Intellectual Property Rights (TRIPS) agreement has already seen a change in the patent laws which have put access to medicines and thereby health care beyond the reach of the masses. In a study published by the journal *Health Affairs*, illness and medical bills caused half (50.4%) of the 1,458,000 personal bankruptcies in 2001. The study estimates that medical bankruptcies affect about two million Americans annually – counting debtors and their dependents, including about 700,000 children. Most of the people who filed for medical bankruptcy were middle class; 56 per cent owned a home and the same number had attended college. In many cases, illness forced breadwinners to take time off work – losing income and job-based health insurance, precisely when their families needed it most. Families in bankruptcy suffered many privations – 30 per cent had a utility cut-off and 61 per cent went without the required medical care.

If this is the condition in one of the countries heralded as the most developed nation in the world, it is a disaster waiting to unfold in India, which is aggressively pushing for privatisation in health care.

Public Health Care in India

Health is a state of complete physical, mental and social well-being. A basic human right and a worldwide social goal, which the countries had pledged to achieve, "health for all by 2000", it remains unfulfilled. Health care covers not merely medical care but also all aspects of a person's sense of well-being, including preventive care and public health. It includes cultural understanding of ill-health and well-being, the extent of socio-economic disparities, reach of health services, quality and costs of care, access to drugs and current biomedical advances. This makes it mandatory for every nation to have a health policy.

The nature of provision of medical health care varies across countries and the socio-economic and political forces within a given society. Countries like Sweden, Britain and India have a history of planned development of health services where the state has played an important role in their finance, supply and management. Prior to the growth of allopathic medicine, medical care, largely based on indigenous systems like ayurveda in India, was in the private hands of households, healers and lay practitioners. It is only in the last decade that privatisation has gained a central place in determining directions in health policy the world over. In Europe at present there are proposals for further privatisation of services in both England and Germany. In Malaysia, there has been systematic and deliberate privatisation of both hospitals and support services in recent years.

India has one of the most privatised health care systems in the world. Though the 1983 National Health Policy (NHP) declared a goal "health for all by the year 2000", the trend of privatisation continues to dominate and grow strongly.

Health care financing is an issue in equity and has two aspects: (a) How much is spent by the government on public health care and on what aspects? (b) How large is the burden of treatment on the poor seeking health care?

In a market economy, health care is subject to three balanced links: the link between (i) state and citizens' entitlement for health, (ii) between the consumer and provider of health services, and (iii) between the physician and patient.

The public health care system in India is deficient. The main reasons are persistent under-funding, insufficient infrastructure (including medicines, trained medical and paramedical staff) and inefficient functioning of district hospitals and sub-divisional centres.

Inadequate funding has plagued the public health sector in India. Public spending (both centre and states) in India on medical and health services is 1.3 per cent of 2004-05 Gross Domestic Product (GDP), and this has barely moved up over the past decade. Total expenditure on social sectors is about 27 per cent of GDP.

Recognising the need to reform the public health care, the NHP 2001 proposed increasing the funding of primary health centres (PHCs) to 55 per cent of the total health budget, the total expenditure for health to 2 per cent of GDP by 2010.

Public spending on health has declined after liberalisation from 1.3 per cent of GDP in 1990 to 0.9 per cent in 1999.

Total health expenditure is 5 per cent of GDP, making public health expenditure a mere 26 per cent of the total health spending. Whereas under five mortality is 95 per thousand in India, Sri Lanka with only 3 per cent of GDP as total health expenditure has an under five mortality of 19 per thousand as its public health expenditure accounts for as much as 45.4 per cent of total health expenditure. Public health spending accounts for 25 per cent of per capita expenditure, the balance 75 per cent being incurred by individual patients, with consequent regressive effects on the poor.

To fill the gap in public health care, the private sector has stepped in. Over the last several decades, there has been an unrestrained growth of independent private medical facilities, which remains urban with polyclinics, nursing homes and hospitals proliferating. The private health sector accounts for 70 per cent of primary health care, and over 50 per cent of all hospital care. In 2001, of all registered hospitals, 73 per cent were in the private sector and 27 per cent in the public sector. In 2002-03, expenditure in the private health care sector was 5.4 times the total public health.

India's public health crisis has deepened with widespread occurrence of HIV epidemic, increasing prevalence of stress related diseases and increasing drug resistance in infections. Lack of access to affordable drugs following the new patent regime has exacerbated the problem. The public health sector is short of hospitals, beds, equipments, medicines, and manpower. Claims of medical negligence and malpractice are frequent. In spite of the risk of infection with HIV, the Government of India recently admitted that 69 per cent of injections administered in public hospitals could be unsafe. Lack of regulation and shortage in supply has led to the proliferation of spurious drugs. Collusion between doctors, medical diagnostic centres and drug suppliers are leaving people to the whims of fate.

Recent Trends

According to government estimates, India's $17 billion health care industry will grow 13 per cent in the next six years. A growing market means larger players entering the scene, that are out to maximise profits and expand coverage, ably assisted by the Indian government. The high tech hospitals are thriving by servicing a small percentage of the population that has the ability to afford high-end medical care at prohibitive costs. This has changed the character of medical care sector.

The most recent trend gaining prominence in India is medical tourism. It is the provision of "cost effective" private medical care in collaboration with the tourism industry for patients from abroad needing surgical or other forms of specialised treatment. Besides, the lure of an exotic holiday thrown in, the price advantage is a key selling point. This process is being facilitated by the corporate sector involved in medical care as well as the tourism industry – both private and public. The genesis of medical tourism lies in the emerging needs of corporate hospitals who are now looking beyond the limited domestic "market" for high cost medical care. Hospitals like Apollo and Escorts are forerunners in this business. Estimates say that foreigners account for 10 to 12 per cent of all patients in top Mumbai hospitals.

The flip side of this high quality care is the unreliable nature and poor quality of overall health services for the poor. The reasons for this are the lopsided, unregulated and largely unmonitored growth of the private health sector. Other deterrents include a lack of political will, inadequate and outdated laws, absence of standards of specification, low levels of consumer awareness and support and lack of concern about conforming to international standards.

Another area of concern is waste management. Without facilities like autoclaves and incinerators, medical waste and discarded organs are just dumped in waste bins and dumping grounds creating a public health hazard with the spread of communicable disease.

Fixing the System

Regulation

Self-regulation systems in India are sadly deficient. The Medical Council has not teethand regulation in the local bodies and the Food and Drug Administration (FDA) is lacking. Under the Charitable Hospitals Act, private hospitals are given concessions on land and liberal tax exemptions against a commitment to reserve free beds for poor patients. Most of the hospitals do not comply, nor are there any procedures to monitor them. If discovered, penalties are deficient.

Accreditation

Doctors practicing in the private sector are some times accused of prescribing excessive, expensive and risky medicines and of adhering to rampant and less than justified use of technology for diagnosis and treatment. An accreditation body would assess hospitals for compliance to standards, ensure proper patient care, and assist in upgrading standard of hospitals through education, training and consultation.

Medical Education

With rapid technological advances, medical education has become more expensive; huge capitation fees are charged for admission. For the qualifying doctors, specialisation is far more attractive as a career option. Most of the 1.2 million qualified doctors in India gravitate towards private practice. The crème gets absorbed in hi-tech hospitals, leaving the public health sector to the lower rungs. These doctors reimburse their medical school fees by earnings squeezed out from patients within a few years into their careers. The public sector and the lower rung nursing homes are left at the mercy of poorly qualified doctors – India has nearly half a million doctors without recognised qualification – from spurious medical schools, untrained para-medicals and quacks. According to a 2001 survey conducted by Indian Medical Association (IMA), Mumbai alone has 10,000 quacks operating in the city.

Affordable Insurance

Insurance is essential for facilitating equitable health care. With the recent opening up of the insurance sector to foreign companies, there is the prospect of two trends. New insurance products will be developed to expand business more by deepening than widening risk covered. The second trend would be to concentrate on urban middle and upper classes and salaried people with capacity to pay. That leaves the poor out in the rain.

In order to be socially relevant and commercially viable, micro-insurance for the poor must aim at a proper mix of health hazards and cover many broad social classes and income groups. Innovative community-based new products can be developed using accumulated experience (for instance Self-Employed Women's Association), so that a minimum core cover can be developed as a model for innovative insurance by panchayats, with reinsurance back-up by companies and government bearing part of promotional costs.

Public-Private Partnerships

Public hospitals suffer from lack of autonomy, inadequate budgets, and faltering and poorly motivated care. The NHP 2002 has in spirit welcomed the participation of the private sector in all areas of health. It is now broadly accepted that the private sector has to step in to provide health care, but the poor remains the responsibility of public sector. With the private health sector concentrating on the urban areas, rural health infrastructure must remain the government's mainstay to ensure wider access to health care for all. There has been talk of public-private partnerships, but it is yet to take concrete shape. Most preventive services can be delivered by downstaging to a public health nurse much of what a doctor alone does now. Community-based health services are another promising area.

Conclusion

Poverty continues to be the biggest stumbling block to good health. Poor health drives the poor into absolute poverty and poverty pushes them back into a poor health status. Health for all, will only become a reality if the State follows certain guiding principles for formulating strategies to ensure health for all. These include recognising the highest attainable standard of health as a fundamental right; strengthening the application of ethics to health policy, research and service provision, and implementation of equity oriented policies and strategies that emphasise solidarity and incorporation of a gender perspective into its health policies.

Health care is essentially for public good and has a far broader meaning than merely the availability of medicine, doctors or nurses. It is also about accountability, standards and regulation. In the current era of globalisation and liberalisation, the government is aggressively promoting the private health care sector. However, unregulated growth in the absence of a proper legislation will mean a continuous infringement on the individual's fundamental right to health. Key social sectors like health and education needs to be delinked from economic policies and also public spending on health care needs to be increased to reach our goal of "health for all".

In the last few decades, an increasing number of countries are realising that health legislation is a potent means of achieving the objective of "health for all". Moreover, a growing awareness among health activists and the urgency to achieve this goal has led to global movements like the People's Health Assembly, which has been replicated across countries like India.

Concrete health rights need a sound legal framework for effective implementation. This framework is based on a combination of many international instruments that impact health rights and national laws and Supreme Court judgments that serve as a basis for human existence. The right to basic health care is recognised internationally as a human right.

4

HIV/AIDS and Socio-Historical Inequality

An Explanation

Vijay Kumar Yadavendu

> The word 'plague' had just been uttered for the first time. Everybody knows that pestilences have a way of recurring in the world; yet somehow we find it hard to believe in ones that crash down on our heads from a blue sky. There have been as many plagues as wars in history; yet always plagues and wars take people equally by surprise.... Our townsfolk were not more to blame than others, they forgot to be modest – that was all – and thought that everything still was possible for them; which presupposed that pestilences were impossible.... They fancied themselves free, and no one will ever be free so long as there are pestilences.
>
> — A. Camus, *The Plague* (1972: 34)

The human immunodeficiency virus/acquired immunodeficiency syndrome (HIV/AIDS), a global pandemic, has decimated the population of Sub-Saharan Africa and disrupted the health and disease care resources of many other zones. Some other Third World countries are seeing the resurgence of old infectious diseases such as malaria and tuberculosis and measles, in addition to new diseases. Indeed, it is a truism that epidemics of infectious diseases have been major contributors to the course of history. Epidemiologic literature is replete with reports of particular investigations, which led to the identification of etiologic mechanisms and their subsequent effects on disease incidence and prevalence in the populations affected. The Black Death (1346-53) and the Great Smallpox (1775-82) are examples of cataclysm, huge and hideous, which shook the entire Europe and North American continents. Public health failed to take lessons from the historical metaphors of epidemics. According to World Health Organisation (WHO), every 60 minutes, 1,500 people die of an infectious disease (Koop, Pearson and Schwarz, 2002). By AIDS Day 2002, HIV/AIDS in Africa had killed 20.4 million and infected 29.4 million people (UNAIDS, 2002).

The dominant biomedical (highly techno-scientific biomedicine) model of public health is clinical, where the public agencies have emphasised individual-focused intervention. Its origin can be traced back to the discovery of the germ theory of disease that emphasised the role of biologic agents and microorganisms in disease causation. In the 1880s, the German bacteriologist Robert Koch proposed a set of requirements to guide researchers in making causal inferences (Carter, 1985 and 1987). Koch's approach demanded that investigative work be carried out in the laboratory, with the investigator isolating the causative agent and studying its presence under the microscope for each case of the disease. The faith in laboratory investigation continued to grow strong with Jacob Henle arguing that infection by minute organisms was a major cause of disease (Rosen, 1937; Shryock, 1972) and Louis Pasteur's demonstration of a living organism as the agent in an epidemic afflicting sick worms, culminating in 1865 (Vallery-Radot and Devonshire, 1901). Studies on infection and contagion in human disease like, tuberculosis, anthrax and leprosy (Vallemin, 1952; Koch, 1996) followed. Finally, in 1882, Koch established a microbacterium as "the cause" of tuberculosis (Goldberger, Wheeler and Sydenstricker, 1918). The mechanical approach to the human being was strengthened by the germ theory of disease where the idea was simple, unitary, and compelling: "one germ-one disease-one therapy". Thus, Henle, Pasteur and Koch and many others can be considered as the symbolic founding fathers of this model of public health.

The new paradigm of health and disease that followed from their work, the germ theory, led to the emergence of a narrow laboratory perspective of a specific cause model (Terris, 1964) relating single agents, one to one, to specific diseases. The focus of epidemiology was restricted to the pursuit of specific agents, singular causes and the means of preventing their consequences (Susser, 1996).

This perspective emphasised on the behaviours that led to infection, is considered appropriate as modes of intervention and prevention. Individuals are the unit of infection and treatment, and therefore the individual became the unit of analysis. Self-care and changes in lifestyles are supposed to be the most important strategies to improve the life span of individual citizens (Navarro, 1976:126). The basic cause of sickness or ill health is located within the individual and not in the system. And the solution, therefore, is intervention, primarily behaviour modification, and not the structural change of the economic and social systems. Thus, broad socio-economic dimensions are systematically excluded from the analysis and, instead, risk is considered largely in behavioural terms. Behaviourism, carried to an extreme, has led to unscientific and reactionary theories such as behaviour modification, which uses unethical and even brutal means to change behaviour. For example, knowledge attitude and practice studies (Rao, 1974:145-379) from India were conducted for introduction or imposition of various methods of contraception. The interventionist concept of motivation was used to change the attitude of the people towards such contraception.

The mundane biological and behavioural factors seem to govern the overall social conditions. It is not intended to suggest here that disease in a population can be understood without reference to biology. The question, however, is what approach one should take: the individual as the unit of study with his or her biology abstracted from social conditions, or disease in populations with biology understood in relation to its social context. The former approach derives from the ideology of individualism, which has at its heart in atomistic individuals of the idealised market, the politics of "market individualism", from which the liberal conception of the social world where individuals are relatively free agents with needs, desires, rights and so on, emerged. In the liberal view social institutions are seen emerging through the decisions and agreements of individuals or groups of individuals. Even knowledge is explained in terms of individual perceivers or thinkers. Subsequently, institutional changes are also explained in terms of relatively free individuals exercising their choice. The social and economic domination exercised by one group of individuals on the other and the consequent class conflict has no place in this theory. The issues of unfreedom, exploitation or inequality are bypassed by drawing upon a naturalistic explanation of social hierarchy. The liberal conception of social hierarchy or inequality can be understood from J.D. Bernal's description of the analogy between social hierarchy and natural order:

> The hierarchy of society was reproduced in the hierarchy of the universe itself; just as there was the pope, bishops, and archbishops, the emperor, kings, and nobles, so there was a celestial hierarchy of the nine choirs of angels, seraphim, cherubim threnes; dominations, virtues and powers; principalities, archangels, and angels (all fruits of the imagination of the pseudo Dionysius). Each of these had a definite function to perform in the running of the universe, and they were attached in due rank to the planetary spheres to keep them in appropriate motion. The lowest order of mere angels that belonged to the sphere of the moon had naturally most to do with the order of human beings just below them. In general there was a cosmic order, a social order, an order inside the human body, all representing states to which Nature tended to return when it was disturbed. There was a place for everything and everything in its place. The elements were in order – earth underneath, water above it, air above that, and fire, the noblest element, at the top. The noble organs of the body – the heart and lungs – were carefully separated by the diaphragm from the inferior organs of the belly. The animals and the plants had their appropriate parts to play in this general order, not only in providing man with necessities, but even more by furnishing him with moral examples – the industriousness of the ant, the courage of the lion, the self-sacrifice of the pelican (Bernal 1969:308).

The social production of health inequality as shaped by liberalism has to be understood in historical context of the emergence of a new capitalist order. The liberal ideology became the *mantra* for the newly emerging bourgeois class at the time of the industrial revolution. This economically empowered bourgeoisie broke free from the fetters of feudalism and a new capitalist order evolved. The new social order was equally capable of extending both freedom and unfreedom and of simultaneously reducing one set of risks to human welfare and survival while increasing others. Thus, what brought emancipation and welfare to one set of people, resulted, at the same time, in a degradation of the quality of life experienced by another set of people. Issues of equity and the responsibility of the state to ensure equity were seen as irrelevant and antithetical to the ideology of capitalism.

Although it has been generally accepted that income inequality leads to health inequality, the causes of income inequality have hardly been in the backdrop of research on health inequality. The focus has simply been on establishing an empirical relationship between income inequality and health or on countering the effects of the former on the latter rather than countering the cause of income inequality. In addition, the primacy of the individual over society meant that the causes of inequality and deprivation were located within the individual and his capability or incapability to reap the fruits of the capitalist system. Foucault traces the transformation (the beginning of which he dates to the close of the 18th century), the very foundation of medical knowledge becomes lodged in the "sovereignty of the gaze" fixed on individual signs and symptoms and then in deep anatomical structures. It is through the observation of individual signs and symptoms that it became "possible to designate a pathological state...a morbid essence... and an immediate cause" (Foucault, 1983: 90). And with the development of pathology, the medical understanding of disease turned even more fully towards "the deep, invisible, solid, enclosed, but accessible space of the human body" (ibid.: 195). Thus, what is known about disease is now a matter of positive knowledge of the individual. What is seen is what is known, and what is known becomes the space for intervention. Locked into a particular way of seeing, an imprisonment reinforced by institutional structures, medicine knows and acts upon disease bounded by an immediacy of perception, which is physical (mechanical, biochemical, visual). In escaping from a nosology of morbid essences, it builds its science and chemical practice on the closed grounds of what becomes, in principle, an observed occurrence within the individual body. Notions of causation are compressed as well, limited to the boundaries of the individual in which disease takes its only meaningful existence. Anything, which cannot be shown to interact with the organism to produce a morbid state, is increasingly excluded. The local space of the disease is also, immediately, a causal space (ibid.: 189). The solution to the problem of disease is directed towards breaking the most immediate cause link. Thus, medical perception pushes causal understanding toward the immediate and local, and solution toward the elimination of symptoms and the restoration of normal signs. As Foucault further states, "the space of the disease is, without reminder or shift, the very space of the organism" (ibid.: 191). Medicine has become "a science of the individual". This is ironic since the problems of ill health and disease in the Third World countries are entirely of a different order, located in hunger, poverty and infection, all of which have social bases. Medicine as a therapeutic or clinical science locates the problem of disease in the individual body (Yadavendu, 2001). Individualism, especially in democratic societies, makes population strategies of prevention an avenue less pursued (Rockhill, 2005). Prevalent public health policy, which is rooted in the liberal philosophy, only serves to perpetuate inequalities. The influence of individualism in public health policy, in the form of "victim blaming" is illustrated taking the case of AIDS.

Blaming Culture of Policy on HIV/AIDS

The AIDS-related policies focused on individual characteristics and behaviours in determining HIV risk is an approach that (Fee and Krieger, 1993) is referred to as "biomedical individualism". The construction of AIDS incorporates distinct views of etiology, prevention, pathology and treatment of disease, each tacitly promoting different conceptions of proper allocation of individual and social responsibility for AIDS.

In the first paradigm, AIDS was considered as a "gay plague" or "gay-related immunodeficiency syndrome" by analogy with the sudden devastating epidemics of the past (Fee and Daniel, 1988). In the second paradigm, AIDS was normalised as a chronic disease to be managed medically over the long term (Fee and Daniel, 1992).

Both the paradigms have tried to capture the effects of the AIDS pandemic, but neither has proved fully adequate. The sudden appearance of AIDS gave meaning to the word pandemic: a disease that spreads is called "spread by leaps" or "metastatic spread", consumes life, and then burns out, leaving devastation in its wake. Epidemiologists, the first scientists to lay claim to understanding the mysterious new ailment, were struck by its seemingly exotic preference for young homosexual or bisexual men, later reported in intravenous drug users, hemophiliacs, and recipients of blood transfusions. They therefore searched for causes in the sexual attitudes, lifestyles and behaviours common to gay men. In the process, they looked for risk factors prevalent in this 'risk group' or 'core' groups and indicated life in the 'fast lane', including 'promiscuity', 'poppers' (amyl nitrate) and anal sex to be the dominant risk factors.

Beyond individual behaviours, pathways by which HIV/AIDS becomes concentrated in a particular racial/ethnic group involve complex processes of economic and social deprivation, socialisation patterns, socially inflicted trauma, targeted marketing of illicit drugs, and inadequate health care (Krieger, 2000). In popular perception, however, all members of the identified risk groups were seen as potentially contagious; from there it was but a short step to stigmatise and discriminate against those risk groups and hold them "responsible" for AIDS. Soon however, the construction of the "other" (as responsible for AIDS) moved beyond social identities to geographical boundaries. Africa came to be regarded as the birthplace of the disease and from there it was supposed to have spread to Haiti, USA and Europe through immigrants, homosexuals and drug users. "The categories of epidemiology and virology have placed a barely invisible cordon sanitaire around minority communities, deviant individuals and the entire continent of Africa" (Patton, 1990).

In 1983, the identification of HIV, the AIDS virus, led to a new phase of the epidemic, in which AIDS was clearly characterised as an infectious disease (Mirko and Grmek, 1990). Once the virus was identified, scientists lost their interest in the social factors accompanying transmission. They instead turned to laboratory studies of the virus and its action within the body in the hope of making new discoveries that would lead to patents, vaccines, and possibly a cure.

The epidemiological perspective that accompanied this kind of biological reductionism concentrated on behaviour modification as the main tool for prevention of the disease. In other words, sexual promiscuity was sought to be controlled. The broader socio-economic context, in which immigrant labour, prostitutes or homosexuals, (considered as potential carriers of the virus) became susceptible to the infection, was completely left out of the sphere of discussion. There is considerable body of descriptive literature from the past decade documenting the general relationship between population movement and HIV/AIDS; there are still relatively few epidemiological data on how different types of population mobility act to increase both individual and community vulnerability to HIV. The transmission and prevention of HIV infection, HIV/AIDS has increasingly become concentrated in poor regions of the world and among poor and marginalised groups in the richer regions of the world (UNAIDS/WHO, 2002). It is historically obvious that the highest incidence rates, regardless of whether the disease is AIDS, malaria, tuberculosis, or heart disease, will be among the poor and stigmatised. The evidence has been consistent since John Graunt's work in seventeenth century England. Moreover, in spite of the accepted linkage between poverty and disease, no concerted effort was made to analyse the role of poverty in the growth and spread of this disease. Hence, the focus on finding a medical cure for the disease as well as the stress on behaviour modification restricted the scope of social epidemiology in public health and put the onus on the individual to save himself or herself from the disease.

The dominant four-fold policy regimes of AIDS, viz., (a) prevention, (b) detention, (c) treatment, and (d) anti-discrimination legislation, also carry the same reductionistic individualistic and mechanistic approach.

The preventive policy of AIDS, for example, is typical of individualism. This policy addresses the public need to stem the spread of the HIV virus. To identify the conception of the individual implicit in this policy domain, the two contrasting approaches to AIDS prevention, viz., the active and passive approach can be considered. Actively preventing the spread of the HIV virus might entail, (i) discovering who all carry the virus and monitoring their behaviour accordingly (i.e., quarantining HIV positive individuals); (ii) passing legislation that threatens to punish HIV-positive individuals who knowingly spread the virus; or (iii) enacting laws that punish non-HIV-positive individuals who commit acts that put them at the high risk of contracting the virus.

The first option, quarantine of all HIV sufferers, has been deemed a practical impossibility given the length of time people are usually sick with the disease. The second option, threatening to punish those who knowingly spread the virus, seems the most feasible and logical of the three. But there are no laws making behaviour conducive to transmission of the virus illegal.

The third option deems as a punishable offence any behaviour that increases the risk of contraction (as opposed to transmission) of the virus.

Given the limitations of an active AIDS prevention strategy, public health policy makers have opted for a more passive approach, one that puts the burden of responsibility on the (non-HIV-positive) individual. The conception of the individual implicit in this kind of policy is existentially strong in that individuals are held responsible for themselves. The state escapes from the responsibility of detecting people with AIDS and passing legislation against the deliberate transmission of the virus. The logic of individualism in preventive policy generally presumes that it is an individual's responsibility to protect himself or herself from acts that may unnecessarily expose him or her to the HIV virus. On the other hand, an individual is entitled to sue for grievance if he or she is exposed to the virus by another individual without prior knowledge. In the first scenario, it is everyman (or woman) for himself. In the second, individuals can only be held responsible for things they know they are getting into, i.e., if one had no prior knowledge that one's partner was HIV positive, then one is not liable for one's high-risk behaviour, regardless of the risk. AIDS preventive policy rests firmly on an ethos of individual responsibility (an existentially strong conception), owing to the absence of organisational capacity necessary to curtail socially deleterious behaviour.

In the case of detection policy, treatment and anti-discrimination law, the same narrow and myopic understanding is reflected. The whole range of AIDS infected patients are clubbed under one fraternity with total disregard to their socio-economic location. Here, individuals are seen as autonomous, sometimes intractable, actors. As argued by several critics, twentieth century biomedical models of public health are typically reductionist; they put primacy on explanations of disease etiology that fall within the purview of medical intervention that narrowly is constructed, focus on disease mechanisms, and view social features leading to disease as being secondary if not irrelevant (Navarro, 1986; Waitzkin, 1983; Terris, 1980).

Proponents of such models may even consider emphasis on societal factors such as poverty or discrimination to be unscientific and polemical. Despite lip service to multi-factorial etiology, they seek parsimonious biomedical causal explanations highlighting the role of one or a few proximate agents, and they generally assume that biomedical interventions, operating on biological mechanisms, will be sufficient to control disease. Some have argued that World Bank structural adjustment programmes designed to stimulate private-sector growth and exports in debtor countries have had a negative impact on HIV/AIDS pandemic by undermining rural subsistence economies, expanding transportation infrastructure, increasing migration and urbanisation, and reducing investment in health and social sectors (Lurie, Hintzen, and Lowe, 1995). The national responses to the spread of HIV/AIDS, for example, the cases of Uganda and Thailand, where epidemic levels of HIV infection have decreased in recent years, are frequently used as "success stories" documenting the pragmatic impact of individual-level behaviour change interventions (UNAIDS, 1998). Though, the discrete causes of these successes are often difficult to identify. But structural-level health policies governing prevention, treatment, and care can contribute to dramatic reductions in HIV/AIDS incidence. For instance, Brazil's national response to the epidemic demonstrated the fundamental importance of social change in preventing the spread of HIV, as much of the widely discussed "Brazilian experience" has been attributed to structural changes and social movements which extend well beyond the scope of individual behaviour change programmes (Parker, 1996; Teixeira, 2002).

There is little place for understanding how behaviours are related to social conditions and constraints or how communities shape individuals' lives. From this perspective, populations and sub-groups within populations – including "risk groups" – consist merely of summed individuals who exist without culture or history. There is no acknowledgement of the fact that when epidemiologists "succeed in identifying populations at risk of disease, it is because these risk groups typically overlap with the real social groups possessing historically conditioned identities" (Krieger and Bassett, 1986). Beyond these measures, the individual is powerless to control disease – provoking environment, be they drugs, air and water pollutants, or food additives, except as he becomes knowledgeable enough to participate in public debate and in support of governmental controls (Knowles, 1977: 80).

This is nowhere more evident than in case of AIDS in poor countries. Although AIDS is identified as primarily a disease of the poor and though there is an understanding that poverty and developmental schemes lead in myriad ways to exposure of specific groups to occupations like prostitution, interventions simply involve a search for medico-technical solutions and behaviour modification of individuals or risk groups.

Conclusion

The focus of the dominant biomedical model of public health has always been on individual responsibility of self-help and self-care. Relegating to the background the larger social, structural, cultural and economic context in which lifestyles are "created", public health policies have continuously emphasised on behaviour modification. There is a tendency to focus on individual responsibility, which promote a "blaming culture". The AIDS policy is one of the best examples of this reductionistic and myopic approach of public health.

Public health, like in other social sciences, cannot be traced without reference to the historical development of political and socio-economic systems. For an equitable and just society a sound public health is vital. Thus, a meaningful discourse on public health of HIV/AIDS with transdisciplinary collaboration and achieving sustainable improvements is part of a political exercise, and the search for an alternative holistic vision must retain its political and social context.

References

Bernal, J.D. 1969. *Science in History*, Vol. 1, Penguin, Harmondsworth, p. 308.

Carter, K.C. 1985. 'Koch's Postulates in Relation to the Work of J. Henle and E. Klebs', *Medical History*. Vol. 29, pp. 353-374.

— 1987. *Essays of Robert Koch*, trans., Greenwood Press, New York.

Fee, E., and Daniel, M. 1988. *AIDS: The Burdens of History*, California, University of California Press, Berkeley.

— 1992. *AIDS: The Making of a Chronic Disease*, California, University of California Press, Berkeley.

Fee, E., and Krieger, N. 1993. 'Understanding AIDS: Historical Interpretations and the Limits of Biomedical Individualism', *American Journal of Public Health*. Vol. 83, pp. 1477-86.

Foucault, M. 1983. *The Birth of the Clinic: An Archaeology of Medical Perception,* Pantheon, New York.

Goldberger, J., Wheeler, G.A., and Sydenstricker, E.A. 1918. 'A Study of the Diet of Nonpellagrous and Pellagrous Households in Textile Mill Communities in South Carolina in 1916', *Journal of American Medical Association*. Vol. 71, pp. 944-949.

Knowles, J.H. 1977. 'The Responsibility of the Individual', *Daedalus*. Vol. 106, pp. 57-80.

Koch, R. cited in M. Susser 1996. 'Choosing a Future for Epidemiology: I. Eras and Paradigms', *American Journal of Public Health*. Vol. 86, pp. 668-673.

Koop, C.E., Pearson, C.E., and Schwarz, M.R. (eds.) 2002. *Critical Issues in Global Health*, California: Jossey-Bass, San Francisco.

Krieger, N. 2000. 'Discrimination and Health', in Berkman L.F and Kawachi, I. (eds.) *Social Epidemiology*, Oxford University Press, New York, pp. 6-75.

Krieger, N., and Bassett, M. 1986. 'The Health of Black Folk: Disease, Class, and Ideology in Science', *Monthly Review*. Vol. 38, pp. 74-85.

Lurie, P., Hintzen, P., and Lowe, R.A. 1995. 'Socioeconomic Obstacles to Roles of the International Monetary Fund and the World Bank', *AIDS*, Vol. 9, pp. 539-46.

Mirko, D., and Grmek, D. 1990. *History of AIDS: Emergence and Origin of a Modern Pandemic*, translation by R.C. Maulitz and J. Duffin, Princeton University Press, Princeton. They have told the story of scientific competition over the discovery of HIV briefly but very effectively.

Navarro, V. 1976. *Medicine Under Capitalism,* Prodist, New York.

— 1986. *Crisis, Health and Medicine: A Social Critique*, Tavistock, New York.

Parker, R.G. 1996. 'Empowerment, Community Mobilization and Social Change in the Face of HIV/AIDS', *AIDS*. Vol. 10 (Suppl.3), pp. 27-31.

Patton, C. 1990. *Inventing AIDS*, Routledge, London, p. 99.

Rao, K.G. 1974. *Studies in Family Planning in India*, Abhinav Publications, New Delhi, pp. 145-379.

Rockhill, B. 2005. Commentary: 'The Message is Rarely Simple: The J-Curve and Beyond', *International Journal of Epidemiology*, Vol. 34, pp. 44-45.

Rosen, G. 1937. 'Social Aspects of J. Henle's Medical Thought', *Bulletin of Inst. History of Medicine*, Vol. 11, pp. 509-537.

Shryock, R.H. 1972. 'Germ Theories in Medicine Prior to 1870: Further Comments on Continuity in Science', *Clinical Medicine*. Vol. 7, pp. 81-109.

Susser, M. 1996. 'Choosing a Future for Epidemiology: I. Eras and Paradigms', *American Journal of Public Health*, Vol. 86, pp. 668-673.

Teixeira, P.M. 2002. 'Programme Implementation and Scaling Up: Barriers and Successes', XIV International AIDS Conference. Barcelona, Spain.

Terris, M. 1964. *Goldgerger on Pellagra Bacon Rouge*, La, Lavisiana State University Press.

— 1980. (Editorial) 'The Life Style Approach to Prevention', *Journal of Public Health Policy*, pp. 5-9.

UNAIDS. 1998. 'A Measure of Success in Uganda: The Value of Monitoring both HIV Prevalence and Sexual Behaviour', *UNAIDS*. Geneva.

—. 1998. 'Connecting Lower HIV Infection Rates with Changes in Sexual Behaviour in Thailand: Data Collection and Comparison', *UNAIDS*, Geneva.

UNAIDS/World Health Organization. 2002. 'AIDS Epidemic Update, December 2002', Joint United Nations Programme on HIV/AIDS, New York.

Vallemin, J.A. cited in R. Dubos, and J. Dubos. 1952. *The White Plague, Tuberculosis, Man and Society*, Little Brown, Boston, Mass., pp. 98-99.

Vallery-Radot, R. and Devonshire, R.L. 1901. *The Life of Pasteur*, trans., London, England.

Waitzkin, H. 1983. *The Second Sickness: Contradictions of Capitalist Health Care*, Free Press, New York.

Yadavendu, V.K. 2001. 'Social Construction of Health: Changing Paradigms', *Economic and Political Weekly*, Vol. XXXVI, No. 29, p. 2791.

II

Health, Disease and Social Structures

5

Tribal Health Problems

Some Social Science Perspectives

B.V. Babu and Y.S. Kusuma

Tribals constitute about 8 per cent of India's population and are spread out mostly in Madhya Pradesh, Bihar, Orissa, Andhra Pradesh, the north-eastern states, West Bengal, Maharashtra and Rajasthan. Altogether, there are 427 tribal communities including 75 primitive tribal groups. Due to multidimensional factors, this population is facing many problems like poverty, illiteracy, difficult terrain, isolation, superstition and inadequate health facilities. Several anthropogenic factors like deforestation, industrialisation, displacement-rehabilitation and socio-cultural transformation processes like diffusion, assimilation, acculturisation and intrusion of the non-tribals to tribal habitats have created a complex change in the tribal life as a whole, and eventually influenced their health and nutritional status. On the other hand, due to geographical reasons, they inhabit very small villages scattered over a large stretch of mountainous terrains. Studies on poverty profiles and estimates from micro-studies show that 62 per cent of tribal groups live below the poverty line (UNDP, 2005). Wide dispersal of smaller habitation with poorer communication facilities results in poor outreach of health care. The general health problems are malnutrition related diseases, parasitic diseases including malaria, diarrhoea, respiratory disorders, etc., and genetic disorders including sickle cell disease, thalassemia, etc. These problems have to be tackled keeping scientific observations and studies on the social structure and cultural practices of these socio-economically as well as technologically backward people. It has been realised earlier, but the irony, is that our planning has not considered the dynamism of tribal eco-system, social milieu and "felt need" of the time. The planning and implementation of effective strategies for redressing the problems of tribal health need a critical appraisal from a social science perspective.

Epidemiological Profile of Indian Tribal Population

An integrated multidisciplinary approach to study the tribal health problems has been adopted by different researchers (Basu, 1986; 1990; 1993; 1994; Basu et al., 1989; Bardhan et al., 1989; Swain et al., 1990; Mohapatra and Das, 1990; Rizvi, 1986; Haque, 1990; Chaudhuri, 1986; Friedman and Somani, 2002, etc.). The data on morbidity, mortality and other health indicators reveal that the health status of tribal population is very poor. These studies have indicated that communicable diseases, genetic disorders (haemoglobinopathies), and nutritional disorders are more prevalent. On one hand, communicable diseases still show higher burden while on the other non-communicable diseases are on the increase despite the poor low nutritional status and higher physical activity in their communities, thus increasing the disease burden. The situation of some of the major health problems is presented hereunder.

Communicable Diseases

Malaria

Due to environmental situation and forest ecology, malaria is a putative endemic disease in the tribal communities since long back. Though the tribals form only 8 per cent of the total population in India, it is estimated that they contribute about 25 per cent of the total number of malaria cases and about 50 per cent of *P. falciparum* (cerebral malaria) cases. Epidemiological data from the endemic belts of the country revealed high *P. falciparum* transmission in forests of India, and the tribal population dominates these areas. Malaria control in these settlements has always been unattainable due to technical and operational problems as well as refracting behaviour of vectors to insecticides and parasites to chloroquine, a commonly used anti-malarial drug. Malaria in India is unevenly distributed. In most parts of the country about 90 per cent malaria is unstable with relatively low incidence but with a risk of increase in cases in epidemic form every 7 to 10 or more years. This depends on the immune status of the population, the breeding potential of the mosquitoes and rainfall being the leading cause of malaria epidemics as it creates high mosquito population. In North-Eastern States efficient malaria transmission is maintained during most months of the year. Intermediate level of stability of malaria transmission is maintained in the plains, forests and forest fringes and predominantly tribal settlements in eight states (Andhra Pradesh, Jharkhand, Gujarat, Madhya Pradesh, Chhatisgarh, Maharashtra, Orissa and Rajasthan). Because of the peculiarities of the transmission in the dynamics in the forests and difficulties in control operations compounded by technical obstacles, this type of malaria has come to be known as forest malaria or tribal malaria requiring specialised malaria control efforts (Pandey, 1996). Thus, malaria is prevailing among almost all forest dwelling tribes and continues to pose an important public health problem not only from the point of its contribution to the country's disease burden but also the economic losses associated with it (Sharma, 1998). The government, through its National Anti-Malaria Programme (NAMP), is undertaking several activities including providing for presumptive treatment to fever cases at each village, presumptive radical treatment at health facilities in high-risk areas, promotion of use of insecticide treated bed nets, use of larvivorous fish in mosquito breeding sites and selective indoor residual spray in high-risk areas. Presently these activities are going under World Bank assisted Enhanced Malaria Control Programme which is in operation in 1,045 malaria hardcore tribal primary health centres (PHCs) of 100 districts covering 62 million population (WHO, 2005).

Leprosy

Leprosy is communicated through intimate and prolonged contact with the patient. Besides, lack of personal and domestic hygiene and overcrowded living are also the causative factors responsible for this kind of disease. Leprosy is prevalent among some tribes of Jharkhand, Chhattisgarh, Assam, Orissa, Uttar Pradesh, Tripura, Gujarat and others. The habits and practices of the tribals and the poor economic condition are responsible for it (Ali, 1994). Similar reports of incidence of leprosy in tribal communities are published (Naik et al., 1999 and Rao et al., 2000).

Tuberculosis

This disease is reported among various tribal groups. The causative factors are nutritional deficiencies, personal hygiene, environmental hygiene, overcrowding and the lack of knowledge of prevention among the tribes. Ali (1994) reported tuberculosis cases among the Kondh of Burlabaru of Phulbani district of Orissa and also among the Kondh of Kurli of

Koraput district. He reported that the poor diet and unhygienic conditions are responsible for their prevalence; and disease communication is due to lack of ventilation and close association with the infected members. Similar reports are available from other tribal areas also (Chadha et al., 2003; Murhekar et al., 2004; Datta et al., 2001; Narang et al., 1999). It is reported from tribal population of Car Nicobar that the prevalence of tuberculosis infection increased significantly between 1986 and 2000 and high risk of transmission of infection is observed on this island (Murhekar et al., 2004).

Venereal Diseases and Human Immunodeficiency Virus (HIV)/Acquired Immunodeficiency Syndrome (AIDS)

The sexually transmitted diseases are reported among the tribal communities of India. Some are of the opinion that their contact with the non-tribals is responsible to some extent for the spread of these diseases. Vyas (1980) reported the presence of syphilis and gonorrhoea among the Bhils of Rajasthan. According to him, the new means of communication and transport facilities have made possible fast and cheap mobility between place of work and place of residence. Swain et al. (1990) reported syphilis of 10 per cent of Desia Kondhs of Phulbani district of Orissa. It is reported that the venereal disease infections is 8.9 per cent of the Santhals of Mayurbhanj district of Orissa (Nandy, 2003).

The rapid spread of HIV/AIDS in rural Indian communities has been attributed to the country's poor health infrastructure, poverty and lack of awareness (Maniar, 2000; NACO, 2003). Despite these indicators, little is known about the risk factors, transmission rates, or the impact AIDS will have in these populations in the future. Traditionally, there has been little research and only a paucity of health-related research conducted among this potentially high-risk vulnerable population (Naik et al., 2005). These communities are geographically distinct; with each tribe having its own unique customs, traditions, beliefs and practices. Even within a particular tribal entity, differences in dialect, health practices, unique customs, values, and traditions are apparent. A recent study among some tribal communities of southern Karnataka revealed that the tribal communities did not have a structured marital system; instead, they practised a form of 'serial monogamy' in which they change partners and remarry every four to five years. Regarding sexual practices, 35 per cent of the respondents reported either pre-marital affairs or extramarital affairs. However, such practices were more common in men compared to women. Furthermore, 20 per cent of the male participants reported having had sex with a commercial sex worker during the period the wife had had a child (ibid.). The tribal community throughout India have remained socially and culturally alienated from the mainstream until developmental and conservation activities in tribal areas forced interactions between them. Displacement of the tribal people of southern Karnataka has led to a complex process of rapid acculturation and loss of cultural identity. As they struggle to maintain their traditional social structure, they must adopt new skills, beliefs, and practices necessary for success in their new environment. During this acculturation process, they have been faced with a myriad of public health challenges complicated by poverty, ignorance, and reluctance to abandon traditional beliefs and practices that would allow them to assimilate successfully.

The high level of poverty, inadequate health resources, ignorance and high-risk beliefs and practices among the tribal communities has contributed to the vulnerability of this population. As such it has created a highly susceptible population for the rapid spread of HIV/AIDS and other STDs as well. Because tribal members are forced to migrate outside of their communities in search for work and increased wages, this may contribute to the spread of HIV/AIDS as many engage in extra-marital affairs, seek commercial sex partners, or are under the threat of sexual harassment (females). While there has been limited scientific research exploring the cultural context of extra-marital sexual behaviours, it is generally noted that in these communities, extra-marital affairs are condoned and widely practiced especially during periods when women are pregnant or nursing or during period of travel for work (Bhattacharjee et al., 2000). This kind of behaviour creates a fertile ground for HIV transmission and spread. The data of Naik et al. (2005) indicate that tribal women are particularly vulnerable for HIV/AIDS in some tribal communities, since many of them commence sexual activity at an early age, and get married early as well. Also, they are in a culture that condones extra-marital sex, and this exposes the women to a particularly precarious situation, increasing their risk for acquiring HIV. It is evident from this study that the Indian tribal community is experiencing a latent phase that is potentially a precursor for an HIV/AIDS epidemic. There is a high prevalence of behavioural risk factors, coupled with ignorance, and inadequate health infrastructure thus creating a potential risk for rapid spread of HIV/AIDS, as well as other related diseases (Naik et al., 2005).

Yaws

It is a non-venereal disease caused by Treponema pertenu reported among the tribals of the Agency areas of Orissa and Andhra Pradesh (Nandy, 2003). Ali (1994) and Chhotray (2003) reported a few cases of yaws in Orissa. High incidence of 7 per cent of yaws is reported among Abhujmarias of Madhya Pradesh (RMRCT, 1994).

Non-communicable Diseases

Progressive aging of the populations, freedom from some communicable diseases and changing socio-economic situations paved the way for increase in prevalence of some non-communicable diseases that are associated with increased life expectancy and altered lifestyle. However, there is paucity of information on non-communicable diseases among tribals. Cardiovascular diseases (CVD) are a major problem in the developed countries and are becoming equally important in the developing countries also. CVD are present in many forms, however, those related to atherosclerosis, rheumatic fever and hypertension comprises the greatest burden among chronic CVD. Also, while these disorders or diseases are declining due to several preventive measures and by the provision of health care in developed countries, they are increasing in the developing countries and often these are perceived to be affecting only the rich within these communities. However, it is clear that as the CVD epidemics mature the burden of CVD shifts to the poorer and less educated sections from the richer and better educated sections. Rising burdens of CVD are now being reported in the poor in several developing countries and as the epidemic advances globally, the poor among the countries and the poor within the countries will become the major victims. A substantial proportion of individuals possess hypertension. Kusuma et al. (2004) reported that nearly one-fifth of the tribal population in Visakhapatnam district of Andhra Pradesh possess different stages of hypertension. This study also indicates that low socio-economic groups are also becoming more vulnerable to the risk of hypertension. Though the prevalence of hypertension in the tribal population is comparatively lower than that in the rural and urban population, but is not at all negligible in these tribal communities whose people were mostly under chronic energy deficiency (CED). Despite this higher burden of hypertension none of the tribal respondents were aware of their blood pressure or hypertension status. Previous studies from India have reported variable hypertension prevalence in tribal communities (Dash et al.,1986; Babu et al., 1996; Mukhopadhyay et al., 1996). Kusuma et al. (2004) found lower prevalence of hypertension among a primitive tribal group and high prevalence of hypertension in an acculturating tribal population and they depict acculturation as a cause for increased blood pressure levels and increased prevalence of hypertension. On other non-communicable diseases such as diabetes and cancers, there are very few specific studies among tribal populations (Tripathy et al., 1979; Sarker et al., 1989).

Genetic Diseases

Genetic diseases particularly sickle cell disease, glucose-6-phosphate dehydrogenase (G6PD) deficiency and thalassemia are observed to occur in significantly high frequencies amongst the tribes. The sickle cell anaemia frequency varies across the tribes. It is reported that sickle cell disease frequencies are very high in certain tribes (25% to 37.7% among the Soligas of Karnataka and Pardhans of Andhra Pradesh respectively). It is estimated that around three children in every thousand births among tribes of Orissa and Andhra Pradesh are suffering from sickle cell anaemia (Babu et al., 2002). Tribals are endogamous social groups and they prefer consanguineous or cross-cousin marriages. This type of marriage perpetuates genetic diseases. It is also estimated based on the crude birth rate and frequency of this deleterious gene that around 700 births are occurring every year with sickle cell disease and also 27,000 sickle cell carriers are emerging every year only among tribal population of Orissa and Andhra Pradesh states (ibid.). Regarding G6PD deficiency, the frequency is about 10 per cent among the Santals, Koya Doras of Andhra Pradesh and Angaminagas, Bhuyan, Juangs and Munda tribals of Orissa. The prevalence is especially high that is, more than 15 per cent among the tribes of Madhya Pradesh, Maharashtra, Tamil Nadu, Orissa and Assam, especially in hyperendemic malarial zones (Basu, 1995). Several reports indicated high prevalence of G6PD deficiency among tribal populations of India (Saha et al., 1990; Rao and

Gorakshakar,1990; Naidu et al., 1995; Reddy et al., 1995; Murhekar et al., 2001, etc.). It is estimated that about 13 lakhs of tribal people in India are suffering from G6PD deficiency (DST, 1990). Thalassemia contributes significantly for the anaemia cases in tribal population. Thalassemia (both alpha and beta thalassemia) occurs in a sizeable proportion of tribal population and has been recorded from all parts of India. Alpha thalassemia is more common in tribal population of Andhra Pradesh, Orissa, Maharashtra, Tamil Nadu, etc. Similarly the beta thalassemia is found in all regions of the country (Balgir, 2000).

Malnutrition

The provision of optimal food and nutrition is an important responsibility of the state towards its citizens. It is redundant to say that healthy people enhance the human resources of a nation, which ultimately contribute to a healthy economy (Gupte et al., 2001). It is known from the literature that the nutritional status of not a single tribe of India can be said to be satisfactory. National Institute of Nutrition (1971) and Planning Commission of India (1980) reported high protein-calorie malnutrition along the rice eating belt. Studies on tribes of Maharashtra and Bihar indicate the deficiency of calories as well as proteins and essential amino acids through major signs of nutritional deficiencies (Chitre et al., 1976). Among the tribes of Assam, high incidence of goitre, angular stomatitis and vitamin-A deficiencies are reported (Gopalan, 1971). Similar reports on tribal malnutrition are reported from Orissa (Mahapatra and Das, 1990; Haque, 1990; Kar et al., 2002), Madhya Pradesh (Basu et al., 1989) etc. It is known from various micro studies that majority of these tribal communities are suffering from various micronutrient deficiency disorders (Nayak and Babu, 2003).

The nutritional problems of tribal communities are full of obscurities and very few comprehensive studies are available on dietary pattern and nutritional status of the communities. Rao (1996) concluded that nutritional status of tribes seems to be influenced by their habitat and socio-economic condition. Due to massive deforestation, the economy of forest resource based communities and eventually their nutritional status are affected badly. Studies of tribals of Orissa have found that an ecological imbalance caused by the rapid deforestation has resulted not only in depleting food resources, but in prolonged droughts, adding to hunger and starvation (Ali, 1992). On the other hand, the people are leaving their traditional food products based on wild plants and animals, and dietary habits in a compulsive situation. The tribal diet is also regulated by certain norms and traditions. For example, the Sauras of Orissa consider drinking milk as a taboo (Singh, 1995). Several tribes on Eastern ghats do not consume milk or milk products such as curd. Similarly, consumption of milk is completely prohibited and eating of egg during the pregnancy is a taboo among Kharias (Roy et al., 1999). Also, due to socio-cultural transformation processes like assimilation they are adopting new dietary practices without understanding its nutritional implication. For instance, under the influence of the Hindu caste society, some communities such as Tana Bhagat of Bihar Gonds of Chhattisgarh region have turned vegetarian (Singh, 1995).

Issues Related to Health Services

Health services in India before independence mainly catered to the needs of armed forces, civil servants and elites. Allopathy with curative bias was promoted (to the neglect of the other Indian systems of medicine), but was inaccessible to the vast majority of rural and tribal people. Though considerable progress and improvements have been achieved in terms of technology and resources, the elite and urban bias orientation has not been changed. The mortality rates constitute sensitive indices of the socio-economic status of a population, and considerably higher mortality rate are noticed amongst the tribe. The percentage of mothers who underwent institutional deliveries are remarkably lower among tribes (17%) than the general population (40.1%). Similar disparity existed for other indicators like percentage of mothers delivered with assistance of doctor (14.5% vs. 37.3%), percentage of mothers received antenatal check-up from doctor (34.7% vs. 56.5%), percentage of mothers taken tetanus toxoid injections during pregnancy (46.4% vs. 72.2%), etc. (NFHS-2, 2000). High rates of under-five mortality, indicate not only the socio-economic status, but also nutritional security among children. The high level of mortality rates among tribes, are due to malnutrition, poor intra-natal care, low birth height, afflictions with vaccine preventable diseases (total vaccine coverage is still only 26.4%), poor socio-economic and environmental conditions accompanied by high levels of female illiteracy and poor personal hygiene (Gupte et al., 2001). The indicators of outreach of health services show a wide gap between the tribals and non-tribals due to lack of "all season approachable roads", urban orientation of the health personal, certain cultural constraints and administrative callousness. When compared with general population (53.3 vs. 40.7 neonatal mortality per 1000 live births; 30.0 vs. 21.1 post-neonatal mortality per 1000 live births; 83 vs. 61.8 infant mortality per 1000 live births; 46.3 vs. 22.2 child mortality per 1000 live births; 126.6 vs. 82.6 under five mortality per 1000 live births) (NFHS-2, 2000). The reasons for lower utilisation of PHC services were apathy of the staff, the status barriers between doctor and the people of low socio-economy group (Zurbrigg, 1984). Discussion on health services will entail descriptions of existing health manpower, infrastructure, nature of their distribution and finally impact of all these on the health status of the people. In India, about 35 per cent of primary health centres are functioning with no doctors (Mukhopadhyay and Choudhury,

1997). The situation is similar in case of paramedical staff, and this manpower shortage worsens the malady in tribal areas further. It is clear that first there is a gross inadequacy of health infrastructure. The PHCs and sub-centres have been so located that the distances to be covered (in these areas this means by foot) average about 272 kilometres and 37 kilometres with the highest going up to 465 and 50 kilometres respectively. Similarly, the average number of villages/habitations that have to be covered by a PHC and a sub-centre are about 73 and 10, with a high of 1,461 and 379 respectively. Thus, though manpower availability purely in terms of ratios do not seem to be adverse, the siting of the facilities, and poor communications, has resulted in making distance and physical access a major barrier for the utilisation of health care services (Rao, 1998). Secondly, the existing infrastructure is poorly manned and thirdly the existing facilities are inadequately equipped with drugs and other supplies. Likewise, as per a detailed survey of the facilities established in the tribal areas, undertaken by the department of family welfare during 1994-95, 66 per cent of the PHCs require repairs to make them usable, 30 per cent have no electricity (affecting vaccine potency), 62 per cent have no labour rooms or water supply (making institutional deliveries impossible), and 19 per cent are located in thatched buts, one-roomed buildings, sheds, etc., forcing the large number of the 16 staff members to be at home (NCAER, 1994). While 80 per cent PHCs have no BP apparatus, virtually none have any weighing machines or blood testing equipment, making antenatal check-ups only notional. Over 50 per cent PHCs have no operation theatre and of the remaining, in 22 per cent the theatres have no equipments and therefore are unutilised.

In the case of sub-centres, which are a 100 per cent centrally funded programme, 87 per cent are in rented accommodation, which in tribal areas would only mean a portion of a thatched hut. Even in the remaining 13 per cent sub-centres, 50 per cent require major repairs and are unoccupied. While 8 per cent of the remaining 50 per cent have some facilities such as examination table, etc., only 1 per cent have water facility and 6 per cent electricity. Based on these findings one can quite safely assume that by and large the sub-centres are non-functioning and only a statistic – the odd ones being those which are located on the roadside villages/growth centres, etc. All these have resulted in the provision of less than optimal services both in quantity and quality. It is unfortunate that 43 per cent pregnant mothers in tribal areas received no antenatal care and nearly 83 per cent of deliveries have taken place at home. All these rates and indicators bear ample testimony to the poor impact of health services provided to the tribal people. The health investment profile of India shows that the investment in health is around 6 per cent of the total GDP. Out of this, only 21.7 per cent comprised the public expenditure, while 78.3 per cent constitutes private expenditure (World Development Report, 1993). It is clear that the private investments never go to tribal areas and the tribal population, who is in need of health care. Also they are unable to avail it due to poverty, poor access and high cost of services. In compulsory situations, these tribals are approaching private health care institutions with huge spendings from their pockets. This out of pocket expenditure leads them to poverty and indebtedness, as they have to sell their produce or borrow money for high rates of interests from money lenders. It seems that poverty causes illness and illness leads to poverty. World Development Report (1993) indicated that India had the lowest (1.9%) government expenditure on health compared to other nations of South Asia like Thailand (8.2%), Myanmar (7.4%), Srilanka (5.2%), Nepal (4.7%), etc. In India, 75 per cent of government health expenditure go to curative in urban areas where 25 per cent of its population live (Durgaprasad, 1997). It is clear that though policy makers and planners have recognised the importance of providing optimum health to the people, the same is not found in health financing and budget allocations in the health sector.

Planning from Community Perspectives

The present-day model of health care services in India had evolved over the last two centuries and these services were first organised by the British administrators, who totally ignored the indigenous belief systems, lifestyles and health care institutions and practices, which formed an organic unity. Instead of building on these foundations and evolving a new system more suited to the life and needs of the people with the help of modern science and technology, they made an abrupt and total change by introducing the western system of medicine in toto. This decision created a wide gulf between the culture and traditions of the people on the one hand, and the health services on the other. It also deprived valuable contributions, which the Indian traditional medicine could have made. This loss is still not made up, not withstanding the recent support to indigenous system of medicine, which is only a marginal effort in this direction (ICSSR-ICMR, 1980). Though there were many modifications that have taken place in health care system and health plans, they were not given specific priority to the hitherto aboriginal people's health problems. The indigenous knowledge system of ethno-medicine and folk healing practices are going to vanish slowly. The health seeking behaviour and health culture of these people are still not free from superstition, primitivism and localism till date. So, after realising the reality of the tribal health problems, it is imperative to develop a rational, logical and realistic approach to tackle the problems of these people. It is essential to examine traditional treatment materials and procedures, and to introduce the scientifically tenable knowledge system along with the modern health services during development of health plans for the tribal people.

Basic Approach to the Model

The objective of the national health policy, which was formulated in 1983, was to attain the WHO's 'Health for All' goal by 2000 AD, by establishing an efficient health care system that would take cognisance of and address the basic needs of all Indians. A coordinated, intersectional equitable, community participation approach using appropriate technology was advocated as a means to achieve the goals of 'Health for All'. Though the national health policy clearly identified the social and health inequalities among the Indian population, no clear plans and strategies are suggested to tackle the vulnerable sections of the population like scheduled tribes. The existing urban-biased, centralised, bureaucratic, over professionalised and the top-down approach of the existing system should be reorganised. The planning has to be democratic, decentralised and participatory. It should be able to achieve the goals set for 'Health for All'. The reproductive and child health policy, which was based on the International Conference on Population and Development (Cairo, September 1994), was launched in India in October 1997. The basic features of this policy are not only strengthening the strategies of Health for All, but also stressing importance of community-need assessment, participatory planning and a decentralised "bottom-up" approach, that is sensitive to people's problems not only at macro level but also at micro or household level. It insists on the provision of quality health care services, and envisages the protection of human rights, promotion of women development, depression of gender disparities, etc.

Integration of Traditional Health Practices

There are many tribal health practices, which are highly beneficial and which can revolutionise treatment process even in modern medicine. The positive aspects of the tribal health culture and scientifically tenable indigenous healing tools and techniques should be identified, documented and utilised along with the modern medicine system. Tribal people believe in folk medicine because it fits in with their culture, ecology and their way of thinking. If they believe in evil spirits and magic, it must be remembered that, it does not pervade their whole life, but also apply to their view on medicine. Attempts must be made to take pains to see that the modern medicine is presented to them in such a way that it is acceptable to them. It can be made possible, when those attempts make them believe that the modern medicine is such a way that it does not contradict their beliefs. Most of the health-care providers complain of differential attitude of the tribals towards the modern medicine. However, this may not be true since several tribal people are approaching modern private health institutions set up by missionaries or private people to seek treatment by spending from their pocket. In addition, the traditional healers can be utilised as health facilitators or mediators to provide better health outreach among the tribals. However, they should be trained on the knowledge of modern medicine. In a tribal community of Koraput district of Orissa, "anganwadi" workers and some literate people, along with health workers were utilised for detecting leprosy cases (Rao et al., 2000). Another study from a tribal area of Andhra Pradesh demonstrated that involvement of traditional leaders in the tuberculosis control programme might improve services as they are major health service providers in tribal areas and are acceptable as treatment providers to patients and public health providers (Banerjee et al., 2004). Similar study from Tamil Nadu concluded that it is feasible to train literate tribal youth volunteers to detect subjects with chest symptoms in the community and thereby cases of tuberculosis, and they can serve as an excellent model for community participation in difficult areas (Balasubramanian et al., 1995).

Reorientation of Health Personnel

It is well known that timely health care services, clean drinking water and sanitation, information and knowledge are not readily accessible to the tribal communities due to several reasons such as living in remote hilly terrains, which takes few houses to reach the health care centre, non-availability of medicines, doctors, etc. When they reach the health centre, attitude of the health care providers towards the tribal people is somewhat negative in the sense that "these tribal people never understand anything, they don't know anything, they don't swallow the medicines even that we give, they want the disease to be cured as soon as they swallowed the tablets, they come only when the condition becomes serious" and so on. On the other hand, what the tribals say is that while reaching a health centre after a long walk, they generally do not find any doctor. If any person is there, they behave indifferently in the sense that the person is not patient enough to listen to or understand their problem, the same medicines (2 white and red tablets) are given for any of the complaints, etc. Ultimately, the health care providers failed to or are failing to create faith and confidence in the tribals, which in turn restrict tribals to go to their traditional healers instead of visiting a health centre. It has been reported that the health personnel are not staying in the tribal areas. The indicators of outreach of health services among the tribals show quite infrequent visits of health workers to their assigned villages (Babu et al., 2001). It has been also reported that tribal people are not coming up to avail the modern health facilities. It is also not merely for the cultural constraints. The attitude and behaviour of staff are not favourable towards tribal people and the health staffs are indifferent towards them (Babu et al., 2000). Banerji (1975) rightly stressed, "because of their urban orientation, rural health workers have a strong distaste for rural life. This distaste is for the entire way of life and not simply for the very poor facilities there. Health workers therefore tend to keep a distance from the population as a whole". The health personnel working in the tribal areas should involve themselves to understand the tradition of folk medicine and they should try to free themselves from ethnocentrism and realise the concept of cultural relativism. In addition to it, the issue of barrier of alienation is important. Hesitation of health staff to enter into some houses to see mothers and children speaks volumes about the kind of post-natal care that will be made available to mothers and their new born babies (Babu et al., 2000). Zurbrigg (1984) identified that apathy of the staff and the status barrier between the doctor and people of low socio-economic group are reasons for low utilisation of health care services. At the teaching level, the curricula should include the scientific ways and values of tribal medicine, by virtue of which we create a process of integration of tribal medicine with modern medicine. To minimise the gulf between tribal communities and non-tribal health personnel, the health personnel should be informed about health culture, health seeking behaviour, food patterns, taboos, etc., of the tribal communities. Also, there is a need to reorient the attitude of health personnel, who work with those communities for community centred attitude. It will also build confidence in the community.

Strengthening of Community Participation

An important factor of sustained improvements in the health status is efficient and sustainable community participation. It is now the time to train people of the tribal communities to create self-help groups and sustainable health services system by utilising the locally available resources. As the community accepts their own people easily and ethnicity and belongingness factors definitely enhance the outreach of health services, educated unemployed youth among the tribals and traditional healers should be given the priority to work as health volunteers among their own community after providing sufficient training. The traditional social institutions like tribal panchayats, dormitories, art groups, clubs, etc., can also be involved extensively in health programmes. Some studies demonstrated the success of involving local youth and traditional leaders in various health activities (Balasubramanian et al., 1995; Rao et al., 2000; Banerjee et al., 2004). Administration and outside organisations should provide technical facilities, support and should play a catalytic role to create congenial environment to bring healthy scenario among the tribal.

Health Communication

As the tribal health culture and health seeking behaviour are not free from superstition and taboos, scientific health education and health awareness programmes are required to bring pivotal change among these so-called primitive people. A recent review of NFHS data on utilisation of antenatal services by tribal people (Chatterjee and Saha, 2000) indicated that "perceived their services unnecessary" and "lack of knowledge on these services" are main reasons for lower utilisation of services. Before undertaking the health education campaigns, the desired behavioural change of the target population should be identified, and all health and communication activities should be targeted to achieve that desired behavioural change, instead of just pouring the information. In addition, the knowledge, attitude, behaviour of community members with regard to general health or to a particular illness/disease should be understood, and that information should be considered during planning of communication strategies. The message should be prepared in local languages or dialects and it should be provided through folk media and folk art, as most of the tribal people are illiterate. The concept of functionalism and symbolism of tribal art and culture should be understood properly and should be utilised in motivating and educating the tribal people. In nutrition education programmes, the people should be encouraged to utilise the locally available and traditional dietary items.

Other Ameliorative Measures

Along with all the above mentioned measures, planning should be based on the economic upliftment of the community for better economic life and to drive away the poverty. Optimal health status is both cause and consequence of the development status. Development per se stands for an improved quality of life through gains in health, education, living standard and higher income (Basch, 1999). In tribal areas, PHCs are the focus of preventive care as well as simple curative case. Mostly in tribal areas, the average distance of PHC is about 30 kilometres. For symptomatic treatment and preventive care, the journey to these health centres is unthinkable in terms of loss of wages and transportation costs. Many of the tribal villages have no roads and public transport facilities. Many studies have shown that the great majority of those who do make use of PHC services came from villages within a radius of only a few kilometres (Chuttani, 1976). Mobile health teams are to be provided for difficult hilly areas. In tribal areas, weekly market centres are the focal point of activity. Each such centre should be provided with a health facility in order to augment the utilisation of health care services (Basu and Mitra, 2001). The health centres are to be well maintained and essential biomedical equipment should be provided at the PHC level according to the needs of people. Screening of risk groups for genetic diseases and genetic counselling are to be offered to tackle the problem of genetic diseases.

Besides the traditional health problems, now these aboriginal people are facing a new problem, that is, their indigenous knowledge system of ethno-medicine as well as folk healing practices are going to vanish slowly but surely. To understand the tribal culture, social structure and their implications on health and illness, the anthropologists and other social scientists have been playing a pivotal role. The social science knowledge should be utilised during development of health plans and implementation of programmes. The health programmes of these vulnerable communities should be designed in a holistic way keeping scientific observation on the dynamism of their bio-social environment. And above all, an integrated programme based on the traditional health practices with modern medicine should be developed to provide health to all at grass-root level. The policy makers should also keep unbiased view on the regional and intercommunity balances to provide 'equity in health'.

References

Ali, A. 1992. Nutrition. In, *State of India's Health,* Alok Mukhopadhay (ed.), New Delhi, Voluntary Health Association of India.

Ali, Almas 1994. Food habits and health status of the Kutia Kondhs and Dongaria Kondhs of Orissa. In, *Pre-agricultural Communities of India;* (eds.) T.N. Pandit and N.K. Das. Anthropological Survey of India, Kolkata, pp. 123-135.

Babu, B.V., Chhotray, G.P., Hazra, R.K. and Satyanarayan, K. 2000. Study on perceptions and interactions of vulnerable groups with the government health services in Khurda district of Orissa. *The Indian Journal of Social Work,* 61: 54-65.

—. 2001. Community perception of a district health system. *Journal of Health Management,* 3: 109-116.

Babu, B.V., Kusuma, Y.S., and Naidu, J.M. 1996. Distribution of blood pressure and influence of subcutaneous fat on systolic and diastolic levels in a tribal population. *Journal of Indian Medical Association,* 94: 289-91, 293.

Babu, B.V., Leela, B.K. and Kusuma, Y.S. 2002. Sickle cell disease among tribes of Andhra Pradesh and Orissa, India. *Anthropologischer Anzeiger,* 60: 169-174.

Balasubramanian, R., Sachram, K., Selvaraj, R., Xavier, T., Gopalan, B.N., Shanmuyam, M. and Prabhaker. R. 1995. Feasibility of involving literate tribal youths in tuberculosis case finding in a tribal area in Tamil Nadu. *Tuberculosis and Lung Diseases,* 74: 355-359.

Balgir, R.S. 2000. The burden of haemoglobingopathies in India and the challenges ahead. *Current Science,* 79: 1536-1574.

Banerjee, A., Sharma, B.V., Ray, A., Kannuri, N.K. and Venkateswarlu, T.V. 2004. Acceptability of traditional healers as directly observed treatment providers in tuberculosis control in a tribal area of Andhra Pradesh, India. *International Journal of Tuberculosis and Lung Diseases,* 120: 248-276.

Banerji, D. 1975. Social and Cultural Foundations of Health Services System of India. *Inquiry 1* Supplement, 12.

Bardhan, A., Sinha, S.K., Gopinath, K. and Brahmbhatt, A.K. 1989. A study of factors responsible for less or no utilization of health facilities among the Bhils of Madhya Pradesh. *PAC Report.* NIHFW, (Mimeo). New Delhi.

Basch, P.F. 1999. *Textbook of International Health* (2nd Edition), Oxford, Oxford University Press.

Basu, S.K. 1986. Genetics, socio-cultural and health care among tribal groups of Jagdalpur and Konta Tehsils of Bastar district, M.P. In, *Anthropology Development and Nation Building,* A.K. Kalla and K.S. Singh (eds.) pp. 87-105, New Delhi, Concept Publishing Company.

—. 1990. Anthropological approach to tribal health. In: *Tribal Demography and Development in North-East India,* Ashish Bose, Tiplut Nongbri and Nikhlesh Kumar (eds.) pp. 131-142, Delhi, B.R. Publishing Corporation.

—. 1993. *Study on fertility and mortality trends among the tribal population of India:* A Review. Monograph, New Delhi, ICSSR.

—. 1994. A health profile of tribal India. *Health Millions.* 2 (2): 12-14.

—. 1994. The state of the art of tribal health in India. In: *Tribal Health In India,* (ed.) S. Basu, pp. 312-349, New Delhi, Manak Publication Pvt. Ltd.

—. 1995. Health status of tribal woman in India. In: *Tribal Health in India,* Ed. by Bhupinder Singh and Neeti Mohanty, pp. 57-92, New Delhi, Inter-India Publications.

Basu, S. and Mitra, K. 2001. Health development of tribal communities of India: need for action research. *Indian Journal of Social Development,* 1: 134-156.

Basu, S.K., Jindal, A., Kshatriya, G.K., Singh, P., Roy, P. and Sharma, K.K.N. 1989. Epidemiological investigation of haemoglobinopathies and allied disorders, nutrition and physical growth trends, health profile, health seeking behaviour and their environmental correlates for promotion of health care among scheduled tribes. *Report of Department of Population Genetics* and *Hum. Dev., (DGHS).* NIHFW, New Delhi.

Bhattacharjee, J., Gupta, R.S., Kumar, A. and Jain, D.C. 2000. Pre- and extra-marital heterosexual behaviour of an urban community in Rajasthan, India. *Journal of Communicable Diseases,* 32: 33-39.

Census of India. 1991. *Census of India (series* - 1). Registrar General and Census Commissioner of India, Government of India, New Delhi.

Chadha, V.K., Banerjee, A., Ibrahim, M., Jaganatha, P.S. and Kumar, P. 2003. Annual risk of tuberculous infection in Khammam, a tribal district of Andhra Pradesh. *Journal of Communicable Diseases,* 35: 198-205.

Chakraborty, A.K. 2004. Epidemiology of tuberculosis: current status in India. *Indian Journal of Medical Research,* 120: 248-276.

Chatterjee, U. and Saha, K.B. 2000. An overview of utilization of antenatal care services among the scheduled tribe of major states of India. *The Anthropologist,* 2: 37-42.

Chaudhuri, B. 1986. Medical anthropology in India with special reference to tribal population. In, *Tribal Health: Socio-Cultural Dimensions,* B. Chaudhuri (eds.), New Delhi, Inter India Publication.

Chhotray, G.P. 2003. Health status of primitive tribes of Orissa. *ICMR Bulletin,* 33: 1-6.

Chitre, R.G. Dixit, M. Agate, V. and Vailekar, V. 1976. The concept of essential amino acid in human nutrition – a need for reassessment. *Indian Journal of Nutrition and Dietetics,* 13: 101.

Chuttani, C.S. 1976. Factors responsible for underutilization in primary health centre: a community survey in three states in India. *NIHAE Bulletin,* 9: 229-37.

Dash, S.C., Swain, P.K., Sundaram, K.R. and Malhotra, K.K. 1986. Hypertension epidemiology in an Indian tribal population. *Journal of Association of Physicians, India.* 34: 567-70.

Datta, M., Radhamani, M.P., Sadacharam, K., Selvaraj, R., Rao, D.L., Rao, R.S., Gopalan, B.N., Prabhakar, R. 2001. Survey for tuberculosis in a tribal population in North Arcot district. *International Journal of Tuberc Lung Dis.,* 5: 240-249.

DST 1990. *Health, drinking water and management of genetic disorder. DST Technical Report Series.* New Delhi, Department of Science and Technology.

Durgaprasad, P. 1997. The nemesis of health care system in India: challenges for the twenty-first century. *Kurukshetra,* XLV: 31-37.

Friedman, M.S. and Somani, J. 2002. Health conditions in the tribal villages of South Bihar: an epidemiologic survey. *Journal of Association of Physicians India.* 50: 1376-1380.

Gopalan, C. 1971. *Nutritional Atlas of India.* New Delhi, Indian Council of Medical Research.

Gupte, M.D., Ramachandran, V. and Mutatkar, R.K. 2001. Epidemiological Profile of India: historic and contemporary perspectives. *Journal of Bioscience,* 26: 437-464.

Haque, M. 1990. Height, weight, and nutrition among the six tribes of India. In, *Cultural and Environmental Dimensions of Health,* B. Chaudhuri (eds.) , pp. 192-206, New Delhi, Inter India Publication.

Historical and Contemporary Prospective. *Journal of Biosciences,* 26: 4(Supp): 437-464.

ICSSR and ICMR Study Group Report 1980. *Health for all – an alterative strategy.* Indian Institute of Education, Pune.

Kar, S.K., Dash, V.L.N. and Babu, B.V. 2002. Nutritional plight of Orissa: an overview. *Man in India,* 82: 143-154.

Kusuma, Y.S., Babu, B.V. and Naidu, J.M. 2004. Prevalence of hypertension among a few cross-cultural populations of Visakhapatnam district, Andhra Pradesh, India. *Ethnicity and Disease,* 14: 250-259.

Maniar, J.K. 2000. Health care systems in transition III, India. Part II. Current status of HIV/AIDS in India. *Journal of Public Health Medicine,* 22: 33-37.

Mohapatra, L.K. and Das, J. 1990. Nutritional eco-systems of Orissan tribes. In, *Cultural and Environment Dimensions of Health,* B. Chaudhuri (ed.), New Delhi, Inter India Publication.

Mukhopadhay, A. and Choudhury, A.R. 1997. *Report on the independent commission on health in India.* New Delhi, Voluntary Health Association of India.

Mukhopadhyay, B., Mukhopadhyay, S. and Majumder, P.P. 1996. Blood pressure profile of Lepchas of the Sikkim Himalayas: epidemiological study. *Human Biology,* 68: 131-45.

Murhekar, K.M., Murhekar, M.V., Mukherjee, M.B., Gorakshakar, A.C., Surve, R, Wadia, M., Phanasgaonkar, S., Shridevi, S., Colah, R.B. and Mohanty, D. 2001. Red cell genetic abnormalities, beta-globin gene haplotypes, and APOB polymorphism in the Great Andamanese, a primitive Negrito tribe of Andaman and Nicobar Islands, India. *Human Biology,* 73: 739-744.

Murhekar, M.V., Kolappan, C., Gopi, P.G., Chakraborty, A.K. and Sehgal, S.C. 2004. Tuberculosis situation among tribal population of Car Nicobar, India, 15 years after intensive tuberculosis control project and implementation of a national tuberculosis programme. *Bull World Health Organisation,* 82: 836-843.

NACO. 2003. *Findings of Behavioral Surveillance Surveys.* National AIDS Control Organization, New Delhi.

Naidu, J.M., Babu, B.V., Yasmin and Devi, S.S. 1995. Genetic polymorphisms of red cell enzymes in tribes of Andhra Pradesh, India. *Gene Geography,* 9: 7-14.

Naik, E., Karpur, A., Taylor, R., Ramaswami, B., Ramachandra, S., Balasubramaniam, B., Galwankar, S., Sinnott, J., Nabukera, S. and Salihu, H.M. 2005. Rural Indian tribal communities: an emerging high-risk group for HIV/AIDS. *BMC International Health and Human Rights,* 5: 1.

Naik, S.S., Thakar, U.H., Phrande, A.M. and Ganapati, R. 1999. Survey of leprosy in unapproachable and uncovered areas. *Indian Journal of Leprosy,* 71: 333-335.

Nandy, S.K. 2003. Study of communicable diseases with reference to the tribal population of India – a review. In, *Dimensions of Researches in Indian Anthropology.* (eds.) Sahay, V.S. and Singh, P.K. p. 232-239, Serials Publications, New Delhi.

Narang, P., Tyagi, N.K., Mendiratta, D.K., Jajoo, U.N., Bharambhe, M.S. and Nayar, S. 1999. Prevalence of sputum-positive pulmonary tuberculosis in tribal and non-tribal populations of the Ashti and Karanja tahsils in Wardha district, Maharashtra state, India. *International Journal of Tuberc Lung Dis.,* 3: 478-482.

National Institute of Nutrition 1971. *Annual Report, 1970-71* National Institute of Nutrition. Hyderabad, Indian Council of Medical Research.

Nayak, A.N. and Babu, B.V. 2003. Tribal health problems: an anthropological appraisal. *Man in India,* 83: 301-313.

NCAER 1994. *Survey of Primary Health Care.* National Council of Applied Economics Research, New Delhi.

NFHS-2 India 2000. *National Family Health Survey (NFHS-2).* Mumbai, International Institute of Population Sciences.

Pandey, G.D. 1996. Highlights of tribal health research under Indian Council of Medical Research. ICMR Bulletin, 26 (3&4): 21-28.

Planning Commission of India 1980. *Report: Sixth Five-Year Plan.* New Delhi, Planning Commission (Government of India).

Rao, D.H. 1996. Nutritional Profile of Indian Tribes. *Nutrition News,* 17: 1-4.

Rao, K.S. 1998. Health care services in tribal areas of Andhra Pradesh: a public policy perspective. *Economic and Political Weekly,* 33: 481-486.

Rao, P.V., Bhuskade, R.A. and Desikan, K.V. 2000. Modified leprosy elimination campaign (MLEC) for case detection in a remote tribal area in the state of Orissa, India. *Leprosy Reviews,* 71: 377-381.

Rao, V.R. and Gorakshakar, A.C. 1990. Sickle cell hemoglobin, beta-thalassemia and G6PD deficiency in tribes of Maharashtra, India. *Gene Geography,* 4: 131-134.

Reddy, P.H., Petrou, M., Reddy, P.A., Tiwary, R.S. and Modell, B. 1995. Hereditary anaemias and iron deficiency in a tribal population (the Baiga) of central India. *European Journal of Haematology,* 55: 103-109.

Rizvi, S.N.H. 1986. Health practices of the Jaunsaris – A socio-cultural analysis. In, *Tribal Health: Socio-Cultural Dimensions,* (ed.) B. Chaudhuri, pp. 85-98, New Delhi, Inter India Publication.

RMRCT. 1994. *Annual Report: 1993-1994.* Regional Medical Research Centre for Tribals, Jabalpur, India.

Roy, R.U., Basu, U., Mukhapadhya, S. and Ghale, S. 1999. Mother and child care among some Kharia community in Similipal area, Orissa. In, *Contemporary Society: Tribal Studies,* (eds.) D.K. Behera and George Pfeffer, pp. 293-309, 3, New Delhi, Concept Publishing Company.

Saha, N., Hong, S.H., Wong, H.A. and Tay, J.S. 1990. Red cell glucose-6-phosphate dehydrogenase phenotypes in several Mongoloid populations of eastern India: existence of a non-deficient fast variant in two Australasian tribes. *Annals of Human Biology,* 17: 529-532.

Sarkar, S., Nagabhushan, M., Soman, C.S., Tricker, A.R. and Bhide, S.V. 1989. Mutagenicity and carcinogenicity of smoked meat from Nagaland, a region of India prone to a high incidence of nasopharyngeal cancer. *Carcinogenesis,* 10: 733-736.

Sharma, V.P. 1998. Fifty years of malaria control in India. In, *Public Health in India - Five decades,* A Commemorative Volume, pp. 76-94, 1, Kolkata, AIIPH and PH.

Singh, B. 1995. An overview of tribal health. In, *Tribal Health in India,* (eds.) Bhupinder Singh and Neeti Mohanty, pp. 17-32, New Delhi, Inter-India Publication.

Swains, S., Jena, S.C. and Singh, P. 1990. Morbidity status of the Kondh tribes of Phulbani (Orissa). In, *Cultural and Environmental Dimensions of Health,* (ed.) B. Chaudhuri, pp. 177-191, New Delhi, Inter India Publication.

Tripathy, B.B., Panda, N.C., Tej, S.C., Patnaik, D.K. and Samal, K.C. 1979. Prevalence of diabetes mellitus among tribal people of Orissa. *Journal of Associations of Physicians India,* 27: 497-503.

UNDP. 2005. Common Country Assessment (CCA) – India. United Nations Development Programme (http://www.undp.org.in/report/POSITION/CCA.htm accessed on 25 November, 2005).

Vyas, N.N. 1980. Cultural background of venereal disease. In *Disease, culture contact and tribals* (eds.) N.N. Vyas and R.S. Mann. The Tribal Research and Training Institute, Udaipur.

WHO. 2005. Malaria situation in SEAR countries: India. World Health Organization, Regional Office for South-East Asia, New Delhi (http://w3.whosea.org/EN/Section10/Section21/Section340_4021.htm, accessed on 25th November 2005).

World Development Report. 1993. *World Development Report - Investing in Health.* World Bank, New York, Oxford University Press.

Zurbrigg, S. 1984. The health care system. In, *Rakku's Story: Structure of III, Health and Source of Change,* Bangalore, Centre for Social Action.

6

Culture and Health Care

An Interface

Madhu Nagla

Man is unique in having cultural environment. This includes all the conditions in which men are born, live, work, procreate and die. Culture as an environment is deeply related to the health of human beings. Human culture everywhere includes patterns of social organisation designed to regulate a particular society, the members can understand the behaviour of most people and they can predict how an individual will react in a given situation. With our knowledge of medicine, it perhaps seems strange that the treatment of diseases among non-literate peoples so frequently calls for praying, wearing of amulets or in consulting an exorcist who recites certain verbal formula in the process of treatment. To many people illness and disease are unexpected events, not controllable by ordinary means. And it should not be overlooked that many members of our own society quite sincerely believe that disease is best cured, whereas epidemics may be controlled by prayer and faith rather than by medical knowledge (Hasan, 1979). Worship of deities, followed by feasting in calamities like epidemics of cholera and exorcist in certain types of illness or going for a holy bath in other places are still practised in folk societies.

Simply defined, a culture is inclusive of the beliefs and customs of a society which have developed in attempting to manage its shared problem, a part of which concern the occurrence of illness and the need for medical treatment (Enos and Sultan, 1977). By analysing the characteristics of culture of a society, we can understand the health care system. First, most of the beliefs and customs are cultural when they are quite commonly shared by the people of the society. We have a majority of cultural traits with beliefs and customs (including those pertaining to health, illness and treatment) shared by a large number of masses of people; and we have numerous sub-cultures, large groups of peoples who share somewhat different cultural beliefs and customs.

The pattern of health care and health institutions differs from society to society and from time to time. The differences depend to a large extent upon cultural views and norms to disease. The medical institutions have a long history and have developed over a considerable time. They have undergone changes with the rise of technology, varying social needs and the pressures of a variety of interest groups of the institutions of human society. Previously, hospitals were centred around religious monasteries and temples. But the modern health services depend on the argument that hospitals should have a community base. The hospital arises out of the needs of the community and it should serve the community with the best. Lewinski-Corwin observes "hospitals have been coexistent with man's settlement in large aggregations, the rise, decay and recrudescence reflect the development of man's culture, social ideals, religious spirit and scientific achievement".

Variations in cultural environment may be noted among the people of two different groups. For example, in North

India, milk is considered to be an important food and is given to growing children, sick and weak persons. In the south, on the other hand, its use is much less (Hasan, 1979). Healing practices as well as ideas regarding disease also vary considerably. Therefore, it is very important for understanding the health problems in relation to the people, their hygienic understanding, attitudes towards diseases, their orientation or action pattern when somebody falls ill and own remedies to cure certain diseases. In view of this, it is desirable for the social scientists to understand and study the health care of the society and the methods of healing which are no less important for a complete understanding of the total way of life (or culture) of people. The study of cultural environment of a community may help the health administration in framing social policies for health and nutrition of the people.

In order to study medicine it is important to keep in foreground the question of whether specific behaviour patterns are universal, reflecting the exigencies of the human situation, or whether they are the special product of configurations of a specific culture. One can assume that the problems which people face and the psychological needs that arise from these problems are everywhere, at least, similar despite difference in theories about the technique of coping with them. Thus, study of our society with respect to an important problem that of illness in the context of different cultural settings is important. The development of conceptual scheme, of course, depends, in part on the availability of accurate descriptions of different systems of medical care, their techniques and functions.

The development of such a conceptual framework, however, has at least two practical consequences. It provides us with a better understanding of our own system of medicine and medical practice. Second, it provides insights into the application of western scientific medicine in non-industrial societies. The present paper deals with the study of attitudes and beliefs towards medicine and medical care systems and organisations in two different settings, i.e., urban and rural setting in Haryana. In all random sample of 104 respondents has been taken equally from the rural and urban settings. The specific objectives are as follows:

- To identify the belief or conception and orientation about health and medical care of the people which influence their attitudes in seeking medical care.
- To understand the importance of food in a cultural context in terms of food habits, serving habits and eating habits.
- To analyse people's beliefs towards causes and treatment of some common diseases.
- To analyse the dimension of rational, non-rational, fatalistic and non-fatalistic pattern in understanding their behaviour for causes and treatment of illness.

The cultural structure of a particular society regarding perception, preference, evaluation and satisfaction shows the pattern of health care. Thus, it becomes imperative to find out personal hygiene, food habits and nutritional status in relation to its culture. How far beliefs, ideas, values and practices are directly related with the phenomenon of health care. The cultural setting of a society influences directly or indirectly people's understanding of the problems of diseases, its treatment, prevention and the pattern of health care. A person's attitudes, daily routine decisions regarding health maintenance, food habits and food serving practices are reflective of efforts on his or her part to maintain or restore himself or herself to his or her normal state. Even when we know how to prevent some illness or to seek medical care for cure of various diseases, the utilisation of such services will depend on the notion people have of health and illness, actions they take in the event of sickness and on their understanding of the etiology of a disease. Thus, the attitude of the members towards disease, health, food and eating habits form the picture of health pattern. The notion about the local medicines which they use during their illness comes under the framework of ethno-medicine. What sort of knowledge people have towards diseases and what do they do to combat these will also be analysed in the present paper.

Conception of Health

Whenever we talk about health care, what comes immediately to our mind is, "What is health?" We have discussed below the elements of normal health as perceived by our respondents living in rural and urban settings. An individual's response to this concept is likely to be influenced by his background and awareness. Since these perceptions are mostly subjective in nature, one has to define these terms normatively. Norms provide standard of adequacy relevant to capacities, state of feeling and biological functioning needed for the performance of those activities expected from the members of a society.

Health, like happiness, is an elusive concept. It has been defined in a number of ways. But none of the different definitions is entirely satisfactory. To answer the seemingly single question: who is healthy? The World Health Organisation, in 1946, defined health as, "state of complete physical, mental and social well-being, and not merely the absence of disease and infirmity". Good health can be experienced positively or negatively, as something tangible or as absence of health related problems. Herzlich (1973) in his study found that "health is to feel in good form, happy content, with a good appetite, sleeping well, wanting to be up and doing; it is to feel well and strong; that's what good health is". A different definition, given from a sociological perspective, comes from the Parsons (1951), who describes health as a state of optimum capacity for the effective performance of valued task. Parsons focuses attention on the social importance of health: healthy individuals are able to function well in order to perform social roles; ill health reduces their ability to do so.

To some respondents of our study, the term 'health' does not connote anything obscure and elusive. The local equivalent for this is *tandurasti* which means right condition of the body. We have observed that health is hardly ever a subject of talk among the people when they gather at public places at their leisure time. We never heard people talking about their health, unless we asked questions on health.

In the present paper, we have analysed the attitudes towards health based on lay conception of health by the respondents. The following composite answers offer an important illustration of how differently these persons reacted to and perceived their health. We recorded their multiple responses in certain categories. The factor which was preferred first, was kept in first response category, and so on. We have taken a number of factors including physical, biological, socio-cultural and environmental, regularity in habits, economic and psychological, but primarily health is identified through physical and biological standards.

Physical

Out of the total number of respondents in the sample, 66 (44%) persons perceived health on the basis of looks, e.g., "handsome or beautiful". Similarly, "a person is healthy who is neither fat nor thin, or bodily fit in terms of height and weight". Some others feel that a healthy persons should have "sufficient amount of energy, stamina, efficiency". Further "sufferings and injuries should have no effect on their body and able to fight if necessary". Lastly, a healthy person should be "fat *(mota),* or well built and bones should be stout".

Biological

As many as 62 (41.3%) respondents considered biological characteristics for good health. A healthy person is one who has no disease in his body and different functions of the organs work properly. Some reacted: "a person is healthy who keeps normal temperature or not suffering from any disease", etc.

Others

Only 6 (4%) people believed that a healthy person is one who can adjust in diverse situations including capable of taking different foods, water at different places. It means that a healthy person should be in a position to adjust mentally and physically in diverse situations. According to them healthy persons are mentally fit, social, extrovert, polite and they are capable of fulfilling their basic needs. Five (5.3%) emphasised that for maintaining good health, a person should have regular habits in eating, exercise, sleep, work and consumption of balanced diet including vitamins and tonics. Some remarked: "a healthy person should not feel tired after doing hard work". Similarly, "person who is able to follow daily routine things like getting up early in the morning, doing exercises, taking bath daily and have sound sleep". Furthermore, some others also said: "a person is healthy who is good at studies and plays, a person is healthy who takes balanced diet and digests it properly". Four (2.7%) persons considered accumulation of wealth for ensuring good health. They conceive "wealth is health" contrary to the common saying "health is wealth". There is no causal correlation between perception of health and economic conditions here. Four (2.7%) respondents feel that for good health one should be happy mentally because mental illness generally leads to physical illness. Hence, the basic characteristics of health are: confidence, satisfaction and absence of worries, etc. These people provided the following responses for their arguments. These are: "a person who has got confidence, satisfaction, no worries, honest", "a person who remains happy and cheerful, has good thoughts in mind", "a person who does not have any fear" and "a person who does not have any inferiority complex", etc. Given the higher per capita income in the field of our study as compared to backward regions, economic variable does not enter into the perception of the people.

Orientation and Health

While analysing the religious aspects of the concept of disease and its causation, Valunjkar and Chaturvedi (1976) state that the basic principle of Hinduism of "Karma and Rebirth" plays vital role. They argue that health and illness are reward and punishment for one's action in previous birth. It reflects the fatalistic attitudes towards health. Dube (1967) in his study of Shamirpath (Andhra Pradesh) finds that "although indigenous herbs and magico-religious practices are still continued in treatment of diseases, the efficacy and utility of allopathic drugs and injections have greatly changed the attitude of people towards modern medicine". This is a move from fatalistic to rationalistic approach of health as people do not merely believe the super-natural causes of disease but also go for modern treatment. We discuss below the beliefs of our respondents in regards to fatalistic and rationalistic approaches of health.

Generally, one comes across two types of beliefs towards medical practices at different cultural levels. First, at the level of primitive or pre-literate people, there is the practice of "primitive medicine", i.e., medicine based predominantly on the supernatural theory of causation of disease and seeking therapy by magico-religious means (Djurfeldt and Lindberg, 1980). At the folk culture level there is "folk medicine" where the theory of illness involves both supernatural and physical therapy. Thus, people of "primitive culture" and "folk culture" have a fatalistic attitude towards their good health. Second, in traditional and modern societies, "traditional" or "indigenous" medicine and "modern medicine" respectively recognise natural rather than supernatural causation of disease. This view reflects the rationalistic attitude towards good health.

To analyse the extent of orientation of different respondents we have divided statements into four broad categories. They are as follows: fatalistic, non-fatalistic, rationalistic and non-rationalistic. The statements like good health is due to "blessings of God", "good deeds of past" "by offering things to God" were identified as fatalistic orientation. The respondents who gave initial priority to these statements are kept in the category of fatalistic orientation, but others, who did not prefer them are classified as non-fatalistic persons. In the same way, we classified respondents with another set of statements like: "health is the result of good nutrition and hygiene", "hereditary factor" and "good medical care" are some of them which reflect rationalistic orientation. This orientation is also analysed in terms of rationalistic and non-rationalistic oriented people. It is very difficult to categorise people in two exclusive categories of rationalistic or non-rationalistic or fatalistic and non-fatalistic, therefore, we tried to give them rank order.

Fatalism and Health

Fatalism is a concept which combines belief in God, attributes of irrational practices such as superstitions or religious prescriptions. The remedy for a disease caused by God is simple: people promise to offer things to God which they like best, for example, their hair, their children, and even if God is not the cause of illness, he may be prayed to help in curing it. Therefore, a person may go to the temple and pray to God for relief from illness. After his ailment is cured he will visit the temple once again and offers prayer to God along with the offerings. Besides, whenever disease is perceived as a result of failure to fulfil obligations to God, the patient will go to temple and try to improve his relations with God. Often a priest prescribes the means necessary to rectify these relations (Djurfeldt and Lindberg, 1980).

Rationalism and Health

Rationalism is a concept which tries to understand the things in terms of scientific perspective, logic or cause and effect relationship. The diseases which are caused by various types of infection and accounts for a majority of deaths and bad health: fever, intestinal infection, tetanus, small-pox, cholera, tuberculosis, cough, cold, diptheria, etc. Most of the diseases are traced as cause of malnutrition, nutritional deficiencies (vitaminosis, anaemia, etc.), aspects of living standard, inadequate public sanitation and hygiene (worms, stomach diseases, skin diseases, eye and ear infection, etc.). A person's good health is also attributed to the hereditary factors as each individual is related to his generation in terms of his physiological constitution of the body. Generally, it is believed that if an individual has a good health, it is attributed to his hereditary factor. Thus, good health is viewed in the rationalistic perspective in view of "good medical care", "good nutrition and hygiene", and "hereditary factors".

Table 6.1

Ranking of Different Factors by the Respondents Which Affect Good Health

Factors Responsible for Good Health	*Rural*		*Urban*		*Total*	
	Mean	*Rank*	*Mean*	*Rank*	*Mean*	*Rank*
Good deeds of past	1.82	I	1.11	V	1.93	VI
Blessings of past	1.56	II	1.62	III	3.18	II
By offering things to God	1.08	V	1.02	VI	2.10	V
Good nutrition and hygiene	1.43	III	1.90	I	3.23	I
Hereditary factor	1.34	IV	1.57	IV	2.91	III
Good medical care	0.82	VI	1.85	II	2.67	IV

Figures in the table represent mean score.

It is apparent from Table 6.1 that people in general give higher preference to the rationalistic factors for their good health as the total mean value of the factors which show the rationalistic dimension weighs more. But if we analyse each factor separately than "good nutrition and hygiene" was ranked in the first position of rank order and "hereditary factor" scores the third position. On further analysis, it is interesting to note that a large number of rural respondents give higher weightage to fatalistic factor as compared to urban respondents. Urban respondents are more in view of analysing good health in terms of good nutrition and hygiene as it stands in the first rank of rank order.

Habits, Food and Health

Anthropologists view eating habits as a whole complex of culinary activities, likes and dislikes, folk wisdom, beliefs, taboos, and superstitions associated with the production, preparation, and consumption of food in a society, as a major cultural category. And, as a major cultural category, they see food impinging on and related to many other cultural categories. Although they recognise that food is essential to life, it is ultimately a physiological phenomenon. Cultural anthropologists at least, are particularly interested in the role of food in culture as an expressive activity that reaffirms social relationships. Sanctions, beliefs and religion, determine many economic patterns, and govern a large part of the daily round of life. In other words, just as medical systems play roles that transcend health and illness, so do dietary and serving customs play basic social roles that transcend more nourishment of the human body. Some of these roles, and cultural characteristics of food as revealed by our respondents are discussed below.

Food Habits and Health

In rural India people subsist on agriculture and the larger part of the diet is obtained from locally produced foods. It is widely recognised that the diet of the people of a particular area is greatly influenced by local conditions of soil and climate, the density of population, extent of urban contacts, religious customs and traditions relating to fasts, feasts and taboo. Richards (1939) has brought out numerous social and cultural factors involved in the dietary pattern of tribal of Northern Rhodesia has shown that the methods of storage, distribution system of production and cooperation, economic incentives or traditional attitudes and values in relation to food stuffs are at the root of special deficiency in diet.

The purpose of a dietary survey which aims at collecting qualitative information on dietary pattern and food habits is to provide information on the views of healthy food. How food is served in the family? Is there any difference between male and female in terms of serving the food? What are the sources of contamination of food? Do they believe in them and what precautions they take to prevent it? Overall satisfaction and dissatisfaction from the food which they are consuming is also recorded. Food habits and eating habits of individuals grow up in practice and eventually become part of culture.

An important aspects of our study is to delineate the factors considered essential for healthy food. A set of factors is considered on the basis of conceptions of healthy food viewed by the respondents. They are asked to give three responses in order of priority. The higher the mean score, higher was the healthy food for the health of the people. It is apparent from the Table 6.2 that people in Haryana considered milk and milk products, fat, *ghee* and green vegetables as more essential for the health of the people than items like pulses, cereals, meat, fish, eggs, fruits, and dry fruits. Moreover, milk and ghee are easily available to rural people. Generally, every family in rural areas have buffalo in their houses and they utilise milk for their consumption and prepare ghee at home. Urban people also keep buffalo in their house for consumption of pure milk and ghee. However, urban people considered green vegetables as an important item of the healthy food as compared to rural people. This is also a substitute for want of milk. Meat, fish, egg are the insignificant in the given responses as a large segment of pcoplc in rural Haryana are vegetarians. Though, fruits and dry fruits are important items for healthy food, the responses are not significant as these are beyond the reach of the lower and middle classes.

Table 6.2

Mean Score of the Items for the Healthy Food Viewed by the Respondents in Descending Order

Items for Healthy Food	*Rural*		*Urban*		*Total*	
	Mean	*Rank*	*Mean*	*Rank*	*Mean*	*Rank*
Milk and milk products	1.19	I	0.97	I	2.16	I
Butter and Ghee	0.92	II	0.54	III	1.46	II
Green vegetables	0.27	III	0.63	II	0.90	III
Pulses and cereals	0.26	IV	0.37	IV	0.63	IV
Fruits and dry fruits	0.02	V	0.24	V	0.26	V
Meat, fish and egg	0.006	VI	0.17	VI	0.18	VI

There is rural-urban difference though slight, in the perception of healthy food. Fat and ghee are considered less important in terms of healthy food, whereas green vegetables are regarded as important items for the healthy food. They consume them in the form of salad also. The significant thing is to notice that non-vegetarianism is not associated with healthy food, as respondents gave least value attached to meat, fish and eggs. It expresses the cultural heritage of the state as such. Thus, it appears that milk and milk products are dominating items of food in the field of our survey. It is not only the items of food which are important for good health, but also the food habit that may influence health. We turn to this below.

Eating Habits and Health

It is the general habit in the rural area that people take their meals twice a day whereas in the urban area they take thrice a day. Those engaged in agriculture go to their fields early in the morning and work there till evening. The general practice is that workers do not carry their food along with them when they go to the field in the morning. In the mid-day any member of the family, especially the female who cooks food, carries it to the fields for the male workers. Sometimes, children also carry food to the fields. The workers eat the food under the shade of a tree and after a while start working again. They prefer to eat hot food because it removes their tiredness. Further, it becomes inconvenient to eat dry *chappati* (which is the staple food in the area) in the absence of curry vegetables. Besides hot *chappati* and onion they take *lassi* for proper digestion.

Persons who live in urban areas and are engaged in service or shopkeeping or business, usually prefer to have breakfast. Breakfast consists of *parotha,* curd, butter, milk, tea, pickle, etc. The combination of these items depends on individual preferences. People for the day time carry their lunch or those who are near to their working places, take their lunch at home. The items in the lunch vary according to their economic condition, choices and suitability in preparation at home.

Tea has become common for both rural and urban folks. People in villages have also started taking tea. They say that it removes tiredness and in the cold season serves as a hot drink. Foods are generally eaten with the help of hands. There is no system of eating food with spoons, knives and forks in the village. However, in urban areas, some families use spoons for semi-liquid meals. Washing of hands is not so common before eating food in the rural as well as in the urban area. But washing of hands is common after eating the food.

The members belonging to Jat caste background, generally, have milk or milk products for breakfast. They do not eat much vegetables at either dinner or lunch but prefer to have milk or lassi or ghee. There is no restriction for children in villages, about how many times they eat in a day. Generally, parents feel that children need eating many times because after playing they often feel hungry. In urban areas, the educated families give the reason that to eat many times a day disrupts the digestive system of children. They, therefore, restrict their children from eating many times. Some people in urban area feed their infants according to doctor's advice.

Food and Nutrition

Adequate diet tends to be thought of in terms of quantity, not quality, of sufficient staple food, not a balance of many foods. Consequently, malnutrition may exist where the potential exists for an adequate diet. To illustrate Hasan (1971) found that in the North Indian village of Chinaura, "people generally believe that it is adequate quantity of food that is important. The idea of quality is restricted to certain food recognised to be strengthening..." No distinction is made between protective and energy producing foods. We have noted the frequent beliefs that children should not be forced to do anything against their will. So mothers rarely force children to eat certain foods. In this way they themselves develop their own taste. Sujatha (2002) in her study of villages in Tamil Nadu finds that variety in food is sought more in those foods that are consumed in large quantities and frequently, and less in those foods that are consumed in lesser quantities and infrequently.

On the other hand, if they force him/her to take that particular type of food, the child will vomit, or may have diarrhoea or pain, etc. This establishes a relationship between unwanted food and illness. Thus, new food is no longer given. Adequate infant nutrition in West Bengal are based on the classification of food as "hot" and "cold". Food classify as *garam* (hot) which include eggs, meat, milk, honey, sugar, and cod-liver oil, are not given to children during hot weather (which lasts during a large part of the year) or when children are suffering from illness classified as *garam* (hot). In all of these ways cultural practices add to the already serious limitations in nutritional possibilities open to poor, village mothers in West Bengal (Jelliffee,1957). The above description of food value shows that the eating habits of rural people are qualitatively different from the habits of urban people. The adult rural people restrict their eating twice but allow children to eat more times, whereas in urban area the frequency of it is more.

There are strong cultural beliefs about the food given to mothers who gave birth to a child. For example, after delivery of a child, energetic (especially fat) food is given. However, there are some families who cannot afford this kind of diet because of their low income. They reduce the quantity and variety. Even though they have knowledge about the types of food necessary at different times for the body, they provide contradictory reasons for not being in a position to arrange the same (Matthews, 1979). Poverty may be a reason for not being in a position to provide desired food at different times.

Perhaps the most widespread of all food classifications, and particularly significant with respect to health, is the "hot-cold" dichotomy. Whatever the local qualities ascribed to each food, the common theme is that through judicious balancing of foods and the avoidance of excessive amounts of heat and cold, health is most apt to be maintained. Thus, in our study, hot food include raw sugar, buffalo milk, eggs, ghee, meat, garlic, etc. It is believed that milk should not be taken with either meat or fish because of the heat produced. Cold food includes leafy vegetables, carrots, and curd.

Food and Satisfaction

Furthermore, respondents of our field are generally satisfied with the availability of food. When we look at the satisfaction from caste-wise distribution among the population we find that as many as 70 (77.77%) Jats are satisfied with the available food, whereas 15 (68.18%) Scheduled Caste and backward caste respondents are not satisfied with the available food. It may be due to their poor economic conditions in comparison to Jats. Education is also a significant variable in interpreting the relationship between educational level and satisfaction from available food. When we move from illiteracy level towards higher educational level, the dissatisfaction starts increasing. That is why, as many as 44 (83.01%) respondents are satisfied with the available food whatever they get, but among the respondents who had highly professional education were dissatisfied with the available food. Thus, there is a significant relationship between the availability of food and educational level. It is due to the fact that educated persons are very conscious and aware of their rights and privileges.

Besides food, proper drinking water is equally important for maintenance of good health. Adequate supply of safe drinking water and sanitary disposal of human excreta are not only essential for the prevention of some of the common diseases but also for the provision of facilities for a decent standard of living. In countries where water supply and waste disposals have been properly attended to, cholera, typhoid fever, and dysentery have almost disappeared. These measures not only affect infant mortality but also check intestinal parasitic infection rate among the adults.

Infrastructural conditions of water supply are unsatisfactory in the areas – both rural and urban; practically water in the city comes from tubewells which were not deeply dug. As such, it contains lots of soil and other dust particles and other contamination. In the village also, people do not prefer to have medicine which purifies the water in the well. They start quarrelling with the health visitor, as to why they have put medicine in their wells as it has destroyed the taste of their water. They say that *lal dawai* (Potassium Permanganate) is not good, rather it is deterring the taste of their water. Pond is also common in the village. To drink a pond water, means to a have a lot of diseases. There is no flow of water and it is exposed to all impurities. So, from all sides, it is not safe for drinking. Animals also come to this pond. They use it for drinking purpose. People wash their animals and clothes here. Thus, it becomes totally impure but still they use it and become victims of poor health. Access to safe drinking water for the high class is high as compared to backward and Scheduled Castes.

Food and Gender

The sex bias in nutrition for the male against female infants, girls and women, has been brought about by several studies. Girls enter into marriage and motherhood from their pre-existing malnutrition and impair their health further. Cultural traditions of intra-family distribution of food rooted in rural areas, compel women to eat last and often eat least both in quantity and quality. The low intake can maintain her health and nutritional requirements in normal time; but during pregnancy and lactation period, such low intake cannot fulfil the additional requirements causing entrenched deficiencies and ill-health.

This is equally true in urban as well as in rural areas. The improved economic conditions in the state is an important reason for satisfaction with the availability of food. Therefore, economic betterment has been a tremendous factor in improving their health, in fact much more than the advancement of medical sciences (Worht, 1963). It is not only the intake of food, but the norms of eating that are also important for good health.

Norms of Eating Habits

In India, the habit of washing hands before and after meals is common among different communities including Hindus and Muslims, although hands are washed simply with water. Besides, this similarity, Hindus and Muslims differ markedly with regard to their eating habits. Among Hindu caste, no two persons eat together out of the common utensils while this is prevalent among Muslims. According to Muslims, togetherness promotes affection and cordial relations among the individuals. That is why, Muslims do not mind eating a thing already eaten partly by another family member while such a practice is not prevalent among Hindus, except that a married Hindu woman usually takes her meals in the same utensil in which her husband has just taken his meals, without washing the utensils. The habit of eating from the common utensils is unhygienic as this may transfer infection from a sick to a healthy individual.

Norms of eating of the food and practices of drinking water is followed by the practice of serving the food among the family members in the family is another norm which is important in understanding the health of the individual.

Table 6.3

Serving of Food Among the Family Members by the Respondents

Norms of Serving Food	*Rural*	*Urban*	*Total*
They do not serve the same food to all members in the family	48 (64.0)	29 (38.6)	77 (51.3)
They serve the similar food to all the members in the family	27 (36.0)	46 (61.3)	73 (48.7)
Total	75 (100.0)	75 (100.0)	150 (100.0)

Figures in the brackets represent percentage.

In our study, 64 per cent rural respondents as compared to 38.6 per cent of urban respondents state that even today the difference is kept in the distribution of food items between males and females in the family (Table 6.3). In overall sample

50 per cent respondents, who do not serve the same food to all family members in the family gave the reasons for the same in the multiple form.

The most important reason for this kind of behaviour is that the males need more energy as compared to females because they work hard (26 or 17.3%), and they are the chief earners in the family (19 or 12.7%). Besides, the work for rural males is tedious as they have to work under the sun in the field (11 or 14.7%). Another reason for providing more food to male is that the male child will continue to stay at home thereby they will support the parents in old age (7 or 4.7%). The common belief that the girls are discriminated against getting food is not substantiated by our data. As we can see from Table 6.4 that hardly one of the 77 respondents has given the reason.

Table 6.4

Reasons for Not Serving Similar Food Among the Males and Females in the Family

Reasons for not serving similar food	*Rural*	*Urban*	*Total*
Males are given more food in the family as their work is hard/males need more energy	13 (17.3)	13 (17.3)	26 (17.3)
Males are chief earners in the family	13 (17.3)	6 (8.0)	19 (12.7)
Boys are given more food as they remain in the same family even after marriage	7 (9.3)	6 (8.0)	13 (8.7)
Males do hard work in the fields	11 (14.7)	–	11 (7.3)
Sons are helpful in old age	3 (4.0)	4 (5.3)	7 (4.7)
If girls are given more healthy food they will grow fast and then early marriage	1 (1.3)	–	1 (0.7)
Not applicable	27 (36.0)	46 (61.3)	73 (48.7)
Total	75 (100.0)	75 (100.0)	150 (100.0)

Figures in the brackets represent percentage.

It is to be noted that about 73 (48.7%) of the respondents do not discriminate between male and female in serving the same food. As such, nearly half of our respondents do not discriminate. Given relatively the better economic conditions, even this amount of discrimination is not expected. Illiteracy of females may also be the probable reason for this.

After discussing the manner, amount, type and distribution of food, we turn to discuss the influence of evil spirits and bad eye on the food. This is an important belief in the rural area, as such it requires attention.

Effects of Evil Spirits and Bad Eyes on Food

A widely accepted belief connected with health and disease is the effect of evil eye. Some individuals including certain animals are believed to be in possession of certain amount of supernatural power. Children are considered to be most susceptible to the effect of evil spirit and bad eye. But it is not confined to them. It is believed that when a child is very beautiful, it is supposed to have a mysterious evil effect on its health. They identify the evil impact when the child suffers from diarrohea, dysentery, develops fever, and cries loudly and continuously and becomes weak within a short time.

In the village, the common observation was that when the child is under the influence of evil eye, he is not taken to physician, because the physician does not know how to cure such evil spirits. On the contrary, the physician ridicules the patient and their relatives when they talk about it. Accordingly, *jhar phook* (blowing and whiffing) is the therapy suggested for such evil spirits.

As many as 52 per cent of respondents have no such belief in evil eye and spirits on the contamination of food. It is relatively higher in urban area (60%) as compared to rural area (44%) (Table 6.5). One can notice that even in a relatively developed society such as that of Haryana, the believers of bad eyes and evil spirits on food persists even today.

Table 6.5

Belief in Evil Spirits and Bad Eye in Contamination of Food

Nativity	*Belief in Evil Spirits and Bad Eye*			
	Never	*With some conditions*	*Always*	*Never*
Rural	33 (44.0)	15 (20.0)	27 (36.0)	75 (100.0)
Urban	45 (60.0)	16 (21.3)	14 (18.7)	75 (100.0)
Total	78 (52.0)	31 (20.7)	41 (27.3)	150 (100.0)

Figures in the brackets represent percentage.

After identifying the belief about the evil spirits in the causation of certain ailments, certain practices about the belief in the evil spirits and bad eyes in relation to the food are also observed. These practices are the product of experiences of generations without any change. It is interesting to note that even among the urban respondents certain bad eye and evil spirits contaminate the food which further results in certain types of illnesses. However, the belief in evil spirits and bad eye is lower among the urban respondents as compared to rural respondents. As can be seen from the Table 6.5 that 60 per cent of the urban respondents as compared to 44 per cent of rural respondents never believe in such practice.

On further analysing the respondents' belief in spirits and bad eye in contamination of food in relation to their educational status, as many as 39 (73.58%) out of 53 illiterate respondents believed in bad eye and spirits in some conditions, whereas among the educated people 31 (77.5%) out of 40 respondents who are graduate or post-graduate or had professional degree were of the opinion that there are no spirits and bad eye as such which contaminate the food, only eight (20.0%) of these people believed that in certain conditions it contaminates the food. Thus, it seems that there is an impact of education on belief in spirits and bad eye.

Respondents' belief in evil spirits and bad eye in contamination was viewed in relation to different caste background. In all majority of the Jats, i.e., 65 (72.22%) and 13 (56.52%) other castes never believed in evil spirits and bad eye in contamination of food. All the backward caste and Scheduled Caste members either believed in contamination of food by evil spirit and bad eye in some conditions or always. Thus, it appears that lower caste people favour these beliefs. It is also surprising to note that all the Brahmin respondents have belief in contamination of food by evil spirits and bad eye in some conditions and always. It may be due to their inherent belief in their cultural moorings or the same socialisation pattern for these traditions.

Privacy and Food

On further probing, the respondents who had belief in evil spirits and bad eye gave multiple answers for the practices of serving the food among their members for avoiding the effect of evil spirits. The most frequent practice observed was to serve the food to their members inside the house where nobody from outside could watch them so that bad eye may not contaminate the quality of food (22 or 14.7%). This belief was confined to the delicious foods only for some respondents. For instance, eight per cent of the total respondents have such a view. Similarly, a tendency was found to hide the food when somebody visits the house. This practice was more prevalent among rural (12 or 16%) as compared to urban (3 or 4%) respondents. It was believed by 13 (8.7%) respondents that milk should not be left in the mouth as it attracts evil spirits. It was also found that one should not count the edible items. This practice was more prevalent among rural respondents (7 or 9.3%) as compared to urban (3 or 4%) (Table 6.6).

Table 6.6
Forms of Special Practices in Serving the Food Reported by the Respondents

Forms of Practices related to Food	*Rural*	*Urban*	*Total*
Food is served inside the house	10 (13.3)	12 (16.0)	22 (14.7)
If somebody comes in the house from outside, then the food is hidden	12 (16.0)	3 (4.0)	15 (10.0)
After drinking milk it is necessary to wash mouth with water	7 (9.3)	6 (8.0)	13 (8.7)
Delicious food is served inside the house	6 (8.0)	6 (8.0)	12 (8.0)
Food served is not counted	7 (9.3)	3 (4.0)	10 (6.7)
Not applicable	33 (44.0)	45 (60.0)	78 (52.0)
Total	75 (100.0)	75 (100.0)	150 (100.0)

Figures in the brackets represent percentage.

Concepts of Disease and Illness

Disease is not purely a bio-physical phenomenon. It cannot be isolated from the socio-cultural milieu. The perception of disease and its cure assumes different dimensions in different societies. Cultural patterns and typical ways of living give substances to the manner in which disease is perceived, expressed and reacted. To some extent, the cultural context defined what conditions are recognised to assess and define the illness conditions (Mechanic, 1978). Interaction of individuals, disease and society is crucial for the total understanding of health and disease phenomena. The interactional aspect of the problem has revolutionised the medical science in modern times. Though the biological malfunctioning is very much responsible for the disease yet its interaction with the socio-cultural matrix cannot be ignored.

Causation of Disease

Disease is a consequence of the interaction between environmental conditions, specific agents and wide variety of aspects of the host. A known agent may or may not produce disease depending on the conditions of the environment and the host. Genetic factors, nutrition, immune mechanism, social roles, stress, personality, climatic and atmospheric conditions, and the like are all made part of a single concept. Tuberculosis is a disease resulting from an attack of the tuberculo-bacillus on the host; that is, the bacillus serves as a necessity but not a sufficient cause for the disease called tuberculosis. It appears that social and psychological conditions may play some part in affecting a person's residence. While it is obvious that crowded conditions and lack of cleanliness lead to the transmission of disease, and equally obvious that poverty may effect nutrition and the probability of receiving treatment when afflicted, it is not as well recognised that the attitudes of men affect their abilities to withstand physical attack. Although we may not understand the cause of a particular disease, changing conditions associated with disease help to control it indirectly.

Matthews (1979) provides classification of diseases, their symptoms, causes, prevention and treatment. The cause for various diseases are due to visits of the Goddess *Mariamma*, dirty surroundings, eating of certain things, infection, hereditary, and so on. For prevention, there is some improvement of knowledge in the service area. Matthews also observes that immunisation is a method of preventing typhoid, measles, whooping cough and tetanus. It is found that allopathic treatment is not taken for diseases which are believed to have a supernatural causes or for which there is no clear allopathic logic equivalent to the traditional concept of disease. It also shows that most of the diseases which have a common cause of the death in small children are treated mainly by non-allopathic methods. We also tried to find out from the respondents on what they feel about the causes for the diseases. We turn to this on Table 6.7.

Table 6.7
Perception of the Causes for the Emergence of Diseases

Factors	*Rural*		*Urban*		*Total*	
	Mean	*Rank*	*Mean*	*Rank*	*Mean*	*Rank*
Adulteration in food items	1.50	I	1.41	I	2.91	I
Stress and strains in modern life	1.42	II	1.40	II	2.82	II
New insecticide and fertilisers	1.38	III	1.28	III	2.66	III
Weak constitution of the body	1.36	IV	1.21	V	2.57	IV
Poor dwelling conditions	1.03	VI	1.27	IV	1.30	VII
New drugs	1.1	V	1.06	VII	1.16	VIII
Industrial pollution	0.82	VII	1.20	VI	2.02	V
New food products	0.81	VIII	0.84	VIII	1.65	VI

(Figures in the table represent mean score)

What are the main causes for the emergence of new diseases in the sample area of study? It is apparent from the Table that respondents considered adulteration in food as the single, most important factor that affects health. Eating wrong kind of food is the most common cause of disease (Matthews,1979). In their study Djurfeldt and Lindberg (1980) stress the lack of food as also the important cause of disease, while common sense gives equal reverse weight, namely too much food. In fact, the effects of scarcity are also the cause of mental illness as Djurfeldt and Lindberg (1980) view: "Having nothing to eat may also produce mental illness. If a man keeps thinking that he is unable to support his children and family, he may get mentally ill".

The second important factor that was rated, include stresses and strains in modern life as the cause for the emergence of new diseases. Modern life has weakened the social relations due to increasing economic interests of the people which create mental problems in the minds of the people. Nowadays, no one is ready to listen the problems of others. If anyone listens to the problem, he exaggerates it rather than solving it.

People believed that the quality of food has gone down due to new insecticide and too much fertiliser in vegetables and cereals. This was rated as the third important cause of diseases. Fourthly, weak constitution does not have power of resistance and hence is susceptible to any outside effects. Therefore, if a person is very weak and thin, he is likely to become a victim of disease than the strong and sturdy person. Sometimes, hard work and under-nutrition and malnutrition form the weak constitution of the body. To strengthen our point we may give the example of observation made by Djurfeldt and Lindberg (1980) as: "there were great health risks both in the paddy fields (hook worm) and in the salt factory (accidents), and the resistance of the workers is low due to under-nutrition".

The fifth set of factors for the cause of diseases was attributed by the respondents to dwelling conditions, that is dirty surroundings or lack of hygienic conditions, e.g., cholera, malaria and scabies. Therefore, bad sanitation and hygiene is perceived as an important cause of illness. Thus, lack of cleanliness leads to illness. Getting soaked by rain is also a frequent theme. It may cause cold, cough and fever.

Moreover, it is also believed that if purgatives are not given regularly that dirt accumulates in the "stomach" and causes diseases (the stomach, intestines and other internal organs are not distinguished). For example, it is said by some to be due to not taking purgatives (Matthews and Benjamin, 1981).

New drugs were rated as sixth important cause for the emergence of diseases. A variety of drugs with different brands, level and name confuse the masses. These drugs are prescribed by the doctors to the patients on the basis of their publicity, availability and accessibility rather than its characteristics of curability. Many a times these new drugs are the causes for the emergence of new diseases when they have side effects or reactions to the body of a patient.

Quite a few respondents mention the importance of environmental sanitation. For example, flies spread diseases. They are nasty, dirty and foul things. Industrial pollution was rated as the seventh important factor of the causes for the emergence of diseases. However, the urban people became much more victims of the industrial pollution as compared to rural population. Environmental factor is more emphasised by urban people than rural.

New food products is also seen as health risk. A variety of new food products seem attractive through advertisement which show their cheap availability, easy accessibility with different gift schemes, high in the quantity. Therefore, the quality of new food products is not good which harms the body of the people. This last point is recognised by the common sense of our respondents.

Medical Beliefs and Practices

Home medicine is literally the medicine of the people. It comprises medical operative beliefs and practices which are, in principle, available to all the members of a society without reference to their incumbency in a differentiated role or achievement in specialised courses of training. In other words, home medicine represents the uninstitutionalised aspects of the medical cultural pattern. Thus, home medication is an analytical category restricted to the use of *gharelu dawa* (traditional or medicine and home made medicinal recipes) and excludes such aspects as *parhez* (restriction) and "rituals". Home medication may be defined as the taking of treatment without consulting a medical practitioner, qualified or unqualified, and may be based on traditional recipes or even modern medicine.

How did they develop? To begin with, it has probably always been the case that people have tried, mostly through trial and error, to cure themselves when they fall sick. Thus, cures which someone reported as effective would tend to remain in practice; as with magic, it is difficult to disconfirm a cure (except under experimental conditions). Folk beliefs are part of the oral traditional, passed on from parents to children, from older generations to the younger; they thus develop the potent sanction of the tradition. Then, too much reliance on natural remedies developed from the close relationship of people to their land, especially in agrarian areas. Consequently, in traditional societies, the common person's knowledge about medicinal plants and herb is frequently extensive. Therefore, we take medicines for prevention as well as for cure. For the people of the sample area it depends heavily on the natural resources around them.

We discus below the treatment of common diseases prevalent in the field of our study. Every culture consists of a vast collection of "recipes" concerning what to do for various ailments. These recipes may involve herbal consciousness, often of a very unpleasant variety; prescriptions concerning rest or activities; prayers, charms, or a combination of these. Quite often, these recipes are loosely related to folk theories concerning disease; they pass on from generation to generation because they are thought to work effectively.

Nevertheless, people are not aware of the emergence of new diseases, their symptoms or causes and treatment as they are not found in earlier societies. Some illnesses and many injuries, however, were believed to require a doctor's attention. This was particularly true for sudden, severe illness or for chronic symptoms that did not respond to home remedies. People with injuries, such as deep cuts, gunshot wounds, broken bones are usually taken directly to a physician for treatment, including anti-tetanus injections. At the same time villagers and urban people had their own names for diseases which do not necessarily correspond exactly to the allopathic system. The most important diseases which are usually experienced by the people are mentioned with their treatment procedure. The causes for certain important diseases are also replied by the respondents. Still some people of both rural and urban communities believe in goddess *Sitla Mata* for visitation and causing measles and chicken-pox. In chicken-pox, their belief is that the disease does not require any treatment except some natural treatment (such as cooling the body or displaying *neem* leaves on the door) and propitating the *Sitla Mata* goddess. In measles and chicken-pox they stop giving treatment and when the downfall comes they simply give some *prasad* (sweet) for presenting to *Sitla Mata*. Thus, immunisation against measles and other diseases is viewed with suspicion, in part because the theory is unacceptable to the populace.

The important point is that knowledge about the preparation and use of these home medication is widespread throughout the community. Everyone seemed to have a favourite recipe for the cure of specific ailments, and there is a great deal of exchanging of information and testimony about the efficacy of various concoctions. The use of these remedies is tied to some pseudo-scientific belief about the causes of diseases. A healthy state is thought to exist when one maintains a balance between "hot" and "cold" forces. Disease and illness occur when these opposing phenomena become unbalanced. Certain things such as food, liquid or even states of nature are described as inherently "hot" or "cold", depending upon cultural definitions. Thus, the general rule is that one should balance the intake of "hot" with something "cold" and vice versa. Similarly, one takes "hot" medicine for "cold" illnesses and so on. The balance concept also extends to body fluids, especially blood. To be healthy, one must maintain a proper balance not only between fluids, but also maintain them in proper amounts and densities. Thus, if the nature of body is cold or in cold season one should avoid food which increases the coldness in the body for example, curd, raddish, lemon, orange, guava, etc.

An anthropological study by Hitchcock and Minturn (1963) in Koholapur (UP) villages describes medical practices being followed in the village and examines the importance of "hot" and "cold" food, the relationship between small-pox, chicken-pox, measles and cholera and particular God-Goddesses, etc. Gould (1957) and Hasan (1967) attempt similar type of studies in Chattisgarh setting. They note a "connection between hot and cold. The physical and temperamental dimensions of human life is also found in occidental civilisations". Home medication includes an enormous range of drugs, potions, balms, salves – both home remedies and patent medicines. Thus, one takes Aspirin or Saridon for headaches, Analgin or Crocin for tiredness and mild fever, fomentation with water, massages for reducing swelling, and put ghee, coconut oil, salt, etc., on burns and insect bites. Home medical beliefs usually contain many prescriptions for special potions and medicines. For example, a natural substance widely used by people in variety of illness is honey. Honey is used as tonic, as a sedative for nervous conditions, as cold syrup, as a medicine for treatment for eye. Honey is also used in folk belief for preventing bed-wetting in sleep, cleaning stuffy nose, and even reducing pain from arthritis (De forrest, 1958). Moreover, it has variety of uses with other substances in different combinations for the treatment of different diseases. In Ayurvedic treatment, usually, many prescriptions of special potions are given for the treatment.

In the area of folk society, Joseph (1958) has described the practices of the Hutterites, which reveal a curious mixture of understanding of cause-effect relationships and beliefs in supernatural causes in obstertic and paediatric fields. For example, there was some suggestions by our respondents that pregnant women are expected to eat special diet such as milk, ghee, and eggs which are rich in protein, calcium and other growth promoting nutrients, and they refrain from certain chores such as heavy lifting which could cause miscarriage. At the same time, they are careful to have "pure" thought to avoid "making" the foetus and they believe that if a mother see mice and rats, her child may have birth marks as found by Eaton in the practices of Hutteries. After the infant is born, certain precautions are followed, such as putting a black thread around the wrist and waist, marking a black point of *kajal* (collyrium) on forehead and also applying kajal in eyes to avoid the evil eye.

Besides the use of drugs, there are suggestions to support various procedures followed to maintain one's health. These procedures include diets, eating healthy food, regular exercise, sleeping with wide open windows, and taking cold showers, etc. It has also been attributed that stomach-ache caused by over eating, indigestion and some intake of unusual food, uncooked or semi-cooked food. The remedies suggested are: to avoid food for sometime, or take light food. Garlic, asafoetida, thymal (*ajwayan*) etc., are suggested for the proper functioning of stomach. The practice of bath with neem leaves, dettol, massages of almond or sandal oil, etc., has also been used for the problem of skin diseases of scabies, rashes, boils, etc. Tuberculosis and leprosy are infectious diseases. That is why they keep distance from the patient of tuberculosis and leprosy. Onions have been widely used for the prevention of *loo* (sunstroke) in hot summer. It is also suggested that the use of turmeric helps in purifying the blood and brightening the colour for face beauty.

The suggestions, are given in the form of sound sleep or rest, or one should go for light entertainment or change of atmosphere to avoid tensions. For some, Yoga exercises are also suggestive methods of treatment for many diseases. Thus, the practices of all these procedures are not only helpful for the physical treatment but also reduce the mental tension of human beings in our society. Nonetheless, these operative traditional beliefs and practices are rationalised in terms of lay person's conception: either one does not have faith in scientific medicine or for want of modern medicine.

References

De forrest, C. Jarvis (1958) *Folk Medicine*, New York: Holt.

Djurfeldt, Goran and Staffan Lindberg (1980), *Pills Against Poverty: Study of the Introduction of Western Medicine in Tamil Village*, New Delhi: Macmillan.

Dube, D.C. (1967), *Adoption of New Contraceptive in Urban India: Analysis of Communication and Decision Making Process*, Ph.D. Thesis, Michigan State University.

Enos, Darryl D. and Paul Sultan (1977), *The Sociology of Health Care: Social, Economic and Political Perspective*, New York: Preager.

Gould, Harold (1957), "The Implications of Technological Change for Folk and Scientific Medicine", *American Anthropologist*, 59 (June), 507-516.

Hasan, K.A. (1967), *The Cultural Frontiers of Health in Village India: A Case Study of Northern Village,* Mumbai: Nanaktala.

—. (1971), "The Hindu Dietary Practices and Culinary Rituals in a North Indian Villages: An Ethno-medical and structural Analysis", *Ethnomediizin*, 1:57.

—. (1979), *Medical Sociology of Rural India*, Ajmer: Sachin Publications.

Herzlich, C. (1973), *Health and Illness*, Academic Press.

Hitchcock, J.T. and Minturn L. (1963), "The Rajput of Kholapur India", in B.B. Whiting (ed.) *Six Cultures*, New York: John Wiley and Sons.

Jelliffee, D.B. (1957), "Socio-culture and Nutrition: Cultural Blocks and Protein Malnutrition in Early Childhood in Rural West Bengal", *Paediatrics,* 20:128-138.

Joseph, W. Eaton (1958), "Folk Obstetrics and Paediatrics meet the M.D.: A Case Study of Social Anthropology in Medicine", in E.Gartly Jaco (ed.), *Patients, Physicians and Illness,* New York: Free Press.

Lewinski-Corwin, E.N. "Hospital and Sanatoria", *Encyclopaedia of Social Sciences,* Vol. VIII, p. 464.

Matthews, C.M.E. (1979), *Health Culture in a South Indian Village*, New Delhi: Sterling.

Matthews, C.M.E. and V. Benjamin (1981), *Changing Health Beliefs and Practices in Rural Tamil Nadu*, Monograph Series, New Delhi: Indian Social Institute.

Mechanic, David (1978), *Medical Sociology*, New York: Free Press.

Parsons, Talcott (1951), *The Social System*, Glencoe Illinois: Free Press.

Richards, A.I. (1939), *Land, Labour and Diet in Northern Rhodesia,* London: Oxford.

Sujatha, V. (2002), "Food: The Immanent Cause from Outside – Medical Lore on Food and Health in Village Tamil Nadu", *Sociological Bulletin*, Vol. 51, No. 1: 80-100.

Valunjkar, T.N. and H.R. Chaturvedi (1976), "Religion and Illness in Hindu Society", *Journal of M.S. University of Baroda,* 25-26:45-52.

Worht, R.M. (1963), "Health in Rural China: From Village to Commune", *American Journal of Hygiene*, Vol. 77: 228-39.

7

Demographic Determinants of Tribal Health in Rajasthan

B.L. Nagda

Tribes are economically backward groups living in geographical isolation. They are food gatherers, hunters, forest-land cultivators, and forest product collectors. Tribes constitute separate socio-cultural groups having distinct customs, traditions, marriage, kingship, property inheritance system and living largely in agricultural and pre-agricultural level of technology. The dependency of the tribes on nature and their impoverished economy affect population growth, literacy, sex ratio, pregnancy procedure and health care practices. The tribal women are the worst-affected mass who are lacking in literacy, employment, nutrition, health and have limited access to economic assets.

Sources of Data

The information and data regarding tribal population of Rajasthan state has been collected through ethno-demographic literature, census, National Family Health Survey (NFHS)-2 and other surveys conducted in the tribal areas of Rajasthan.

Population Size and Growth

According to 2001 census, Rajasthan has a tribal population of 70,97,706, which forms 12.56 per cent of the total population of the state. The population has grown at a rapid rate during last nine decades and at an almost flooding rate during the last four decades. During 1901 the total population in the state was 103 lakhs, which rose to 565 lakhs in 2001.During the decades 1961-71, 1971-81 and 1981-91 the growth rate of tribal population in Rajasthan was 35.33 per cent, 34.46 per cent and 31 per cent respectively. During these periods the growth rate of tribal population has decreased. The growth rate of tribal population was reported 29.8 during 1991-2001. It is higher than the growth rate of total population of the state (28.33).

Distribution of Tribal Population

According to census 2001 about 71 lakhs or say about 12.56 per cent of the entire population of the state belongs to Scheduled Tribes. The highest concentration is noticed in Banswara and Dungarpur districts where their proportion to total population of the districts comes to 73.47 per cent and 65.84 per cent respectively. Other districts with higher proportion are Udaipur (46.34%), Sirohi (23.39%), Sawai Madhopur (22.47%), Bundi (20.25%), Chittaurgarh (20.28%) and Baran (21.13%). Looking at the dispersal pattern of tribal population of the state in various districts in terms of absolute number, it is observed that the highest proportion (17.75%) of the total tribal population is residing in Udaipur district followed by (15.29%) in Banswara, 10.16 per cent in Dungarpur, 5.81 per cent in Jaipur and 8.39 per cent in Sawai Madhopur districts. As a matter of fact, these five districts together contribute more than half of the state's total tribal population. Other districts have very low proportions, the lowest being 0.08 per cent in Bikaner district. The districts, which have less than one per cent of the state's total tribal

Table 7.1

Percentage of Scheduled Tribes In Rajasthan

Name of District	*Total*	*Rural*	*Urban*
Ganganagar	0.34	0.17	0.97
Bikaner	0.26	0.19	0.38
Churu	0.51	0.48	0.57
Jhunjhunu	1.93	2.24	0.73
Alwar	8.06	8.98	2.39
Bharatpur	2.31	2.63	0.98
Dhaulpur	4.59	5.47	0.39
Sawai Madhopur	22.47	25.97	3.27
Jaipur	7.92	11.82	3.28
Dausa	26.34	28.75	5.96
Sikar	2.65	3.09	1.02
Ajmer	2.30	3.06	1.19
Tonk	11.89	14.53	1.04
Jaisalmer	4.85	5.11	3.44
Jodhpur	2.82	3.12	2.29
Nagaur	0.22	0.23	0.16
Pali	5.40	6.29	2.20
Barmer	5.87	6.24	2.59
Jalor	8.43	8.66	5.55
Sirohi	23.39	27.13	7.98
Bhilwara	9.02	10.35	3.54
Udaipur	46.34	55.97	5.65
Rajsamand	12.82	13.85	5.24
Chittorgarh	20.28	23.47	3.03
Dungarpur	65.84	69.77	15.89
Banswara	73.47	78.83	9.44
Bundi	20.25	23.76	3.58
Kota	9.60	16.18	3.15
Baran	21.13	24.47	2.49
Jhalawar	11.90	13.47	4.02

Source: Census of India, 2001, Rajasthan Census.

population, are Ganganagar, Churu, Jhunjhunu, Sikar, Ajmer, Jaisalmer, Jodhpur and Nagaur (Table 7.1). The population profile of the tribes varies from the general population situation.

Sex Ratio

Sex ratio is the number of females per thousand males. Sex composition of a population is an indicator of the socio-economic and health conditions of males and females. The sex ratio of tribal population (944) was higher than the general population (922) of the state. It shows no sexual discrimination at the time of birth in the tribes. Table 7.2 shows that there are 16 districts where sex ratio of tribal population is 900 females or less per 1,000 males. Eleven districts observed sex ratio in between 900–950 and five districts reported sex ratio of 950 or above females per 1,000 males.

Table 7.2

Districtwise Sex Ratio of Tribal Population, 2001

Sex Ratio	*Districts*
900 and less	Ganganagar (880), Bikaner (817), Churu (884), Alwar (878), Bharatpur (868), Dholpur (834), Swai Madhopur (876), Jaipur (897), Dausa (894), Karoli (854),), Jaisalmer (869), Hanumangarh (868), Nagaur (854), Barmer (885), Bundi (880), Kota (885)
900 – 950	Jalore(903), Jhunjhunu (929), Pali (926), Sikar (923), Ajmer (925), Sirohi (953), Bhilwara (939), Baran (918), Jhalawar (916), Jodhpur (918), Tonk (915)
950 and above	Udaipur (985), Rajsamand (968), Chittorgarh (967), Dungarpur (1028), Banswara (983)

Source: Census of India, 2001, Rajasthan I Population Totals.

It is observed that those districts having higher concentration of tribal population had higher sex ratio. More than half of the tribal population of the state is residing in the five districts, viz., Udaipur, Dungarpur, Banswara, Jaipur and Sawai Madhopur. Bhil and Mina constitute about 95 per cent of the total tribal population. Bhils mainly live in southern districts of the state where sex ratio is more than 950 females per thousand males whereas, majority of Mina concentrate in Sawai Madhopur and Jaipur districts. The Mina tribe is socio-economically well off, having sex ratio similar to general population of the respective districts (Advani and Nagda, 1997).

Tribal Culture and Fertility

Ethno-demographic characteristics of tribes bring out wide variation in the level of fertility within the community. It is mainly because of variation in social, cultural and economic practices. The socio-cultural practices vary from one tribe to another; the tribes are still illiterate and engaged in their traditional occupations. Nagda (1988) reveals that factors like traditional religious systems, value of children, polygamy, remarriage, bride price and poor literacy pave the way for high fertility among the tribes. The average living children of Bhils was 6.7 followed by Christian Bhils 6.2 and Bhagat Bhils 5.4. The age at effective marriage of boys and girls was 18.2 and 17.4 years respectively. More than 50 per cent of the Bhils live in nuclear family consisting of five to six members. Almost all mothers are illiterate. Marriage is usually solemnised after the couple has had the opportunity to know each other intimately over number of months. Divorce is granted easily on grounds of adultery, carelessness in the upkeep of the house, etc. (Nagda, 1992). The results of National Family Health Survey, (NFHS-2) India, Rajasthan indicate the silent issues of fertility pattern of tribes as evident in Table 7.3. About 12 per cent women were currently pregnant and mean number of children ever born to ever married women in age 45-49 was 5.72. More than half of mothers had three and more live births. The median age at first birth was reported to be 19.4 years. Tribal women produced 4.31 children during their reproductive life but they want only

2.7 children. Tribes considered on an average 2.9 children as ideal in their family. The tribal maintain sufficient space between births of two successive children. Median interval since previous birth was 29.5 months. It shows that tribes are aware about adverse implications of rapid growth of population.

Table 7.3
Fertility Indicators of Tribes of Rajasthan

Indicators	*Value*
Percentage of currently pregnant women	12.4
Mean no. of children ever born to ever married women age 45-49 years	5.72
Percentage of third and above birth order of children	55.0
Median age of first birth women in age group 20-49	19.4
Total fertility rate	4.3
Wanted fertility	2.7
No. of children considered as ideal	2.9
Percentage of women wanted at least one son	97.0
Median months interval since previous birth	29.5

Source: National Family Health Survey (NFHS-2) India, Rajasthan, 1998-99.

Level of Mortality

Like fertility, mortality was also higher among tribes in comparison to general population of the state. Table 7.4 reveals that among the tribes 58 births per 1,000 live births do not survive the first month of life, about 37 infants die in between age of one month to 12 months and 95 out of 1,000 infants die before reaching their first birthday. Child mortality (1–5 years) was calculated to be 155. The major causes of infant and child mortality in tribes were acute respiratory infections, fever, diarrhoea and anaemia. It is suggested that for reduction in mortality, especially infant mortality, existing infrastructure of health and medical facilities should be improved and Reproductive and Child Health (RCH) Programme should be popularised more among them through modern and traditional methods of motivation and communication.

Table 7.4

Mortality Indicators of Tribes of Rajasthan

Indicators	*Rate*
Neonatal mortality rate	58
Post neonatal mortality rate	36.7
Infant mortality rate	94.7
Child mortality (1-5 years) rate	155

Source: National Family Health Survey (NFHS-2) India, Rajasthan, 1998-99.

Health Scenario of Tribal Women

Health is the state of complete physical, mental and social well-being and not merely the absence of diseases or infirmity. In Rajasthan, and particularly in the tribes of the state, health status of women is poor and the number of pregnancy related deaths in the tribal areas is higher in the state. The maternal mortality rate in the state is higher in comparison to the country as whole. Malnutrition is widespread among the tribal girls and women. Women have equal rights to enjoy the standard health services, but in reality, women are different and have unequal access to basic health services. The awful poverty, lack of nutritious food and safe drinking water, lack of sanitation and hygienic accommodation, hostile life create problem of health among the women in tribal areas. The early child bearing, miscarriages and multiple pregnancies create serious health hazards for women. Reproductive and sexually transmitted diseases affect the possibility of cancer and AIDS.

The World Bank (1993) estimated that 5 per cent women suffered from domestic violence at the global level. One of the causes of HIV, cancer, tuberculosis and cardiovascular diseases is violence during the reproductive age of women. Over half a million women die every year due to pregnancy related complications. The demographic and health statistics of women prove that health conditions of Indian women are not equally good as men. Maternal mortality and sex selective mortality rate is also higher in the country. Women in India contribute 53 per cent of all hours worked while men contribute 31 per cent. Girls are less likely to be vaccinated and receive medical care when needed than boys. The average nutritional intake for women in India is only 1,400 calories daily while requirement is approximately 2,200. About half of the women suffer from anaemia and two-third suffer from gynecological diseases in India. The likelihood of women dying during pregnancy or childbirth in India is one in 18 as compared with one in 9,850 in Northern Europe (Kalia, 2001). The main factor of violence is the inequality between men and women and discrimination faced by women in their day-to-day life. The violence against women can be conceptualised as an issue of power and social control over women. Nagda (2001) conducted a community survey of 230 women in the tribal areas of Rajasthan and found that among tribal women, 62 per cent women were physically beaten by their husbands at least once a month. Majority (83%) of females reported was verbally abused by their husbands, in-laws and other family members at least once a week. About 39 per cent women suffered mental and physical tortures in the family. Sometimes in extreme forms of violence, the victim may be killed. In the tribal community, divorce and sexual abuse is very common. The unplanned pregnancy, symptoms of sexually transmitted infections (STIs) were more common among wives of the abusive men, especially sexually abusive men who used force. Violence against women includes violence that occurs within the family or within the community in general. Further Nagda (2001) reported that more than two-thirds of the tribal women were abused by their husband, having fights regularly in evening and being insulted, taunted and criticised. The violence among the tribal women was higher in those who work as labourers alone, in comparison to those who work with their husbands. The wives of non-worker, alcoholic and smoker husbands had suffered 45 per cent more from domestic violence as compared to those with working husbands. Majority of the wives who suffered the domestic violence had also suffered many health hazards like Reproductive Tract Infection/Sexualy Transmitted Disease, depression, anaemia, blood pressure, somatic disorders and broken family, etc. In the poor family, main cause of violence against women is their poverty and lack of education. It was further found that frequencies of beating wives with sticks are more in nuclear family than that of the wives in joint family. Violence affected women can have fatal consequences, inducing suicide, homicide and maternal mortality. Violence against women has a major impact on women's physical and mental health and affects their sexual and reproductive health, unwanted pregnancy, the transmission of STIs/HIV, low birth-weight babies, forced abortion and sex selective abortions.

Socio-cultural Issues of Health

Every culture, irrespective of its simplicity and complexity has its own beliefs and practices concerning disease and evolves its own system of medicine in order to treat diseases in its own way. Tribals practise different type of diagnosis and treatments during illness of a person. In tribals, interference of supernatural agency is particularly strong in context of health and disease. The different deities and spirits are connected with various types of disease. The tribal communities have specific gods for treatment of diseases, calamities, treatment of diseases of cattle, snake-bite, dog-bite and so on. All these deities have their own respective sphere and field. The tribal priest is known as 'Bhopa' whose services are sought after, to find out the cause of illness. The Bhopa worship the deities when epidemics and diseases are there in the village, he offers a sacrifice at the sacred place (Devra). He is mainly entrusted with the benevolent deities. Bhopa controls the malevolent deities. The dependency and belief on Bhopa are often responsible for the non-acceptance of modern medicine. The traditional approach established faith and assurance in the patients while modern medicine lacks it. The Bhopa shares the common cultural beliefs and practices of the patients, naturally they have more faith in them. Bhopas (traditional healers) occupy prominent place in the treatment of diseases. If the reason of illness is identified as evil-eye, sorcery or witchcraft, the tribals always would call their Bhopa instead of consulting a doctor, as they strongly feel that the doctors are quite helpless against such evil forces which can only be counteracted by Bhopa (Nagda, 1992). In tribal community, illness and the consequent treatment is not always an individual and familial affair, but the decision about the nature of treatment may be taken at the community level. In case of some specific diseases, not only the diseased person but also the total village community is affected. Health and treatment are very much connected with the environment. The traditional health care system and treatment are based on their deep observation and understanding of nature. The Tribal healer use, different parts of plants not only for treatment, but also for population control. This knowledge can be fruitfully utilised in a wider context.

Nutritional Status of Tribal Women

Tribes are generally fond of non-vegetarian food but they cannot afford it due to their poverty. Body mass index (BMI) can be used to assess both thinness and obesity. The BMI is defined as the weight in kilograms divided by the height in metres squared (kg/m^2). The mean BMI for women in Rajasthan is 19.9. About 40 per cent of Scheduled Tribe women had BMI below 18.5, indicating higher nutritional deficiency among tribal women. More than half (58%) tribal women and 80 per cent of children were suffering from anaemia (NFHS-2). In tribals, problems of malnutrition are due to poverty, illiteracy, lack of nutritional food, health education of the parents and family food habits. Unsanitary environment and unsafe drinking water create a problem of diarrhoea, dysentery, parasitic infections and skin diseases. There are several traditions prevailing among tribes about food intake by pregnant and lactating mothers. The pregnant mother is prohibited to eat ghee, oil seeds, groundnuts, curd and hot foods. Lactating mother is given several types of herbal products and gum with ghee to eat. It is believed that during pregnancy, rich foods containing ghee and fat is injurious to health of womb and after the delivery it is good for the health of mother as well as child. The tribal people of southern Rajasthan, specially Kathodi and Garasia, believe that during pregnancy use of forest foods and animal foods are good for health of mother and child. Kathodi women eat monkey meat during delivery (Nagda, 1996).

Health Care

Ante-natal and post-natal care is one of the indicators of health status of children as well as mothers. Results of NFHS-2 show that 58 per cent tribal mothers were not provided with antenatal care during their pregnancy. They stated that it is not necessary and not customary. About 42 per cent of mothers were given two doses of tetanus toxide injection and 36 per cent were given Iron Folic Acid (IFA) tablets. About 86 per cent deliveries performed at their home and three-fourths of deliveries conducted by 'Dais' and other untrained persons (Table 7.5). Initiation of breast-feeding immediately after childbirth is important because it benefits both mother and infant. As soon as the infant starts sucking the breast, the hormone Oxytocin is released, resulting in uterine contraction that facilitate expulsion of the placenta and reduce the risk of postpartum haemorrhage. It is also recommended that the first breast milk should be given to child rather than squeezed from the breast and discarded, because colostrums provides natural immunity to child. Few mother (3.7%) started breast-feeding within one hour of birth and 74 per cent of the mothers' squeezed first milk from breast. It is suggested that mother should be educated about importance of feeding of first milk.

Table 7.5

Health Care Indicators in Tribals of Rajasthan

Indicators	*Percentage*
Women received ante-natal care	42.0
Received two injections of TT	42.0
Received IFA tablets	35.8
Home delivery	86.0
Delivery conducted by Dais and others	76.0
Children immunisation	
Three doses of DPT	15.7
Three doses of polio	31.5
Measles	19.0
One dose of BCG	39.7
One dose of vitamin 'A'	12.9
Complete vaccination	10.3
Started breast feeding within one hour of birth	03.7
Mother squeezed first milk from breast	73.8

Source: National Family Health Survey (NFHS-2) India, Rajasthan, 1998-99.

Immunisation of children is concerned, about 16 per cent children were given three doses of DPT, 31.5 per cent three doses of polio, 19 per cent of measles, and 13 per cent one dose of vitamin A. The complete immunisation of children was only 10.3 per cent among the tribes.

Delivery Procedure

The tribals believe that when the menstrual period is delayed by a month, women are assumed to be pregnant. She does not take Mahua liquor. There is no restriction on her daily routine work. The delivery (*japa*) is conducted in a hut called *jopada.* The hut is cleaned and pasted with cow dung in advance. The pregnant women go to the hut when labour pain starts. In case of any problem, during the pregnancy, they call traditional Dai of the community. Elderly ladies of the community help in conducting the delivery. The naval cord is cut by mother herself with the help of a bamboo strip, knife and stone. They prefer to cut the umbilical (naval) cord with a bamboo strip because it is more safe from infections (Nagda, 1992). After cutting the umbilical cord, the stump is tied and mahua oil is applied. The mother is given a small quantity of mahua liquor and water mixed with *haldi* (turmeric) and *gur* (jaggary) for drinking for about two days after delivery. They think that these drinks will bring out all harmful substances from the body of the mother. Mothers are advised to avoid sour foods and pluses because they could adversely affect health of the mother and the child. The coloustrum is squeezed out of breast and the baby is breast fed after one day of delivery. The child is breast fed upto 2-3 years. The supplementary food is given to child after 5-6 months. They do not stop breast-feeding during the sickness of the child.

Health Services

Health care system obviously becomes a major component towards the better quality of life of the people. Health care means looking after the people's health in health centre. The health centre is an institution for promoting the health and welfare services in an area under the direction of health personnel under one roof (Paswan, 1994). In tribal areas, 3,000 population served by a sub-centre and 20,000 population have one PHC. Whereas, for general population, a sub-centre serves 5,000 persons and 30,000 population served by a PHC (Government of India, 2001). In tribal areas, the situation is actually worse than the figures indicate because, deficiencies in modern equipment and medical supplies. The effectiveness of doctors in tribal area is less than the areas of total population.

Indigenous Practices of Birth Control

The tribal is an ancient social community. Since long they have the knowledge about indigenous methods of birth control. They use several types of forest products and *jadibuties* (herbals) for controlling the birth as well as removing the sterility. They thought that traditional methods of birth control are easily available with no side effects. The family welfare practice among the tribes is very ancient as a part of their cultural practices. For removing the unwanted pregnancy, they use boiled water of bamboo pills, old gour, leaf of adhatoda, vasica (adusa), clove basil, carsia, black-pepper, *sunth* and thymol. This mixture can be used at any time during the pregnancy but it is believed that if it is used within three months of the pregnancy, it will not be harmful to the health of the mother. The tribals also know the treatment of permanent and safe method of birth control. For permanent method they use juice of *gurbell*, seed of castor and citron, mixing it with gour and give it to the women for 15 days with water. During this period a woman has to take some precautions such as to avoid use of milk, ghee, sour things, and is allowed to take only roti of barley with mung dal without chilies and salt. For maintaining space between two children, they use boiled water of cottonseeds, cannabis sativa seeds (*ganja*) along with picrorhiza (*kutki*). This mixture has to be taken by the female every month for four days after the menstruation period. They even know the herbal treatment for the cure of infertility. In this treatment they use roots of Appamarga plant, seeds of Nagkeshar, steam of Shatawari plant and dry leaf of Sisham and Banyan tree. All these are to be ground together in the form of powder and prepare tablets, dry them at a cool and dry place.

The sterile woman has to take tablets twice in a day with milk of cow for the period of three months. Tribal people also know the treatment of choice of birth. For birth of a son they use Shivlingi seeds with milk after two months of pregnancy. They believed that this herbal treatment is very effective for those women who want birth of a male child. Nagda (1992) stated that among tribals few local healers have knowledge about the herbal medicines and they do not want them to be exposed. They generally keep it a trade secret. The tribal Dayees know these medicines but they also keep it secret. Table 7.7 shows that 29 per cent of currently married women use any method of birth control. About one-fourth of the women use any modern method of birth control. Female sterilisation was more popular among tribes. The need for family welfare was 18 per cent. It is almost same for limiting and spacing methods. About 71 per cent of the women were not using any method of birth control. About 2 per cent women were using traditional methods of birth control.

Table 7.7

Practising Birth Control Methods among Scheduled Tribes in Rajasthan

Indicators	*Percentages*
Current use of family planning methods	
Any methods	29.3
Any modern method	26.5
Female sterilisation	21.8
Male sterilisation	1.0
Not using any method	70.7
Needs of family welfare	
For spacing	8.9
For limiting	9.1

Source: National Family Health Survey (NFHS-2), India, Rajasthan, 1998-99.

Summing up

In tribal areas, there is lack of the physical and manpower infrastructure facilities in the fields of health and family welfare. There is no proper link road between the tribal villages and health centres. Tribals are economically hand-to-mouth. The tribals feel that without money treatment is not possible, hence they always depend on their traditional healer and Bhopas. The entire development programme in tribal areas is running separately. There is no integration between different departments of development. The health centres are not functioning properly due to lack of staff, building, equipments and inadequate finance. The number of health and medical institutions available is entirely inadequate to serve even minimum needs of their health.

References

Advani, M., and Nagda, B.L., (1997), *Sustainable Development and Tribal Population in Rajasthan, Sustainable Development in Tribal and Backward Areas*, Indus Publishing Company, New Delhi.

Census India, (2001), Population Totals, Rajasthan (Floppy Records).

Govt. of India (2001), "Rural Health Statistics in India", Rural Health Division, Ministry of Health and Family Welfare, New Delhi.

Kalia, Anil, (2001), "Investing in Women's Health: The Only Solution", *Social Welfare*, No. 47, Central Social Welfare Board, New Delhi.

National Family Health Survey (NFHS-2) India, Rajasthan 1998-99 (2001), International Institute for Population Sciences.

Nagda, B.L., (1988), "Socio Cultural Mores and High Fertility among Tribals in Banswara", *Social Welfare,* No. 11, Central Social Welfare Board, New Delhi.

—, (1992), *Social Correlates of Fertility*, Himanshu Publication, Udaipur.

—, "Symptom of a Social Malaise", *Social Welfare*, No. 4–5, Central Social Welfare Board, New Delhi.

—, (1996), "Good Nutrition of Healthy Mothers", *Social Welfare,* No. 7, Central Social Welfare Board, New Delhi.

—, (2001) "Population and Reproductive Child Health in the Tribes of Rajasthan", Monograph, Population Research Centre, Sukhadia University, Udaipur.

Paswan, B., (1994), "Spatial Dimension of Health Facilities in Bihar, Population and Development in Bihar", B.R. Publishing Corporation, Delhi.

World Bank, 1993, "World Development Report, 1993: Investing in Health", New York.

8

Tribal Health in India

Tribhu Nath Dubey and Supriya Seth

The word 'tribe' denotes a group of people living in conditions characterised by low level of social and economic development. It is a social group with territorial affiliation, which practices endogamy and has no or little specialisation and differentiation of functions. It is culturally distinct with the other tribal or social groups existing in the region. It has its own distinct dialect, traditions and religion. Ancestor and nature worship and magic characterise its religion. A headman or a chief controls the activities of the group. These tribal groups inhabit widely varying ecological and geo-climatic conditions (hilly, forest, tarai, desert, coastal regions, etc.) in different concentrations throughout the country and are distinct biological isolates with characteristic cultural and socio-economic background (Basu, 1993). They live very close to nature and their livelihood heavily depends on their natural surroundings and its vagaries. As a subsistence economy, they exhibit "hunting or food gathering", "pastoralist", "shifting cultivation" or "settled agriculture stage", depending on their stage of social and economic development. In India they are known as earliest settlers as evident from the vernacular noun, "Adivasi" used for them.

According to the Census of 1991, there are about 67.76 million persons (excluding Jammu and Kashmir) belonging to Scheduled Tribes in India. These constitute 7.95 per cent of total population of India. In Rajasthan, according to 1991 Census, there were 54,74,881 tribal people, which constitutes 12.44 per cent of the total population of the state. In Rajasthan, these are mainly residing in Udaipur, Banswara, Dungarpur, Jaipur and Sawai Madhopur districts. Meenas are numerically the Dominant Group, followed by Bhil, Garasiya Sahariya, Bhil-Meena, Damor and Damariya.

In India, today, tribal groups are most marginalised social groups. The colonial rule in India, Government laws regarding forests and land ownership (see Sarin, 2005), big developmental projects in tribal areas effecting their displacement, lack of literacy and also to some extent their own inward looking tradition bound social set-up have contributed together to their marginalisation. In independent India, various special programmes and provisions (constitutional and legal) with strong positive intent have not been ameliorative to their condition.

Health is one of the most important index of social development. Health is defined by WHO as a state of complete physical, mental, and social well-being and not merely the absence of disease or infirmity. In essential sense health denotes lack of morbidity. Health depends on biological as well as social dimensions. Therefore, one finds high level of morbidity particularly of communicable/infectious type among infants, children and women (Shariff and Sudershan, 1996). It is also true for socially and educationally disadvantageous groups and communities including tribes. Poor hygiene and contaminated drinking water cause most of communicable diseases (biggest cause of morbidity) (ibid.). It is also caused due to specific life-condition of the communities. Economic backwardness, social underdevelopment, low levels of education, persistence of therapeutic superstition, low level hygiene and use of contaminated water makes the tribal communities the worst victim in this respect.

Review of Literature

Though health is one of the prime concerns of our time as it is one of the basic contributors to the development of human resources of any country, the scanning of literature reveals that there is a major gap regarding comprehensive study of tribal health in India. There are scattered efforts in this respect contributed through articles in various journals by researchers, health professionals and activists. Basu (1993 and 1994) has discussed the tribal health scenario and health status of tribal women with all India regional variations. There are reports regarding genetic disorders specifically pertaining to tribal groups in India (Kate, 2000; Basu, 1994 and Ramachandran, 2000). Shariff and Sudershan (1996) provide some important educational and health indicators which provide insight in comparison with the health and educational status of non-tribal communities in India. This paper gathers issues from these scant and scattered literatures along with the data provided by Prayas, Chittorgarh.[1] The data provided by Prayas (2005) provides very useful insight in the tribal health status of the backward area of South Rajasthan. The available literature suggests there are a number of issues, general as well as specific, concerning the tribal health status in India which has common as well as region specific problems and it is in urgent want of sound national policy and strong intervention.

The State and the Tribal Health

On September 6, 1978, the Alma Ata Declaration envisaged "Health for All" by AD 2000. The declaration includes commitment of governments to consider health as a fundamental right, giving primacy to expressed health needs of people, community self-reliance and community involvement, coverage of entire population, effective use of traditional systems of medicine and use of only essential drugs amongst others (Banerji, 2005).

India as one of the 134 signatory countries of the declaration (Phadke, 2003) set "Health for All", as a national goal. The Supreme Court of India has also opined that Indian citizens have a right to basic health care because it is associated with the Fundamental Right to life with dignity (ibid.). Due to Government's commitment to Alma Ata declaration and its efforts towards its realisation people's access to modern medicine has generally improved but it has serious limitations. Banerji (2005) opines that due to acceptance of Sokhey Sub-committee (1948) of National Planning Committee and Bhore Committee (1946) recommendations, the primary health care (PHC) in newly independent India was very near to Alma Ata Declaration on Public Health Care. However, there have been some serious gaps between the policy commitment and their implementation. But post-1982 health policies of India, according to Banerji (ibid.), have undone the good work of the past due to ill-conceived, badly formulated, techno-centric vertical programmes and promotion of "selective primary health care". An Independent Commission on Health in India (1997), set up by the Voluntary Health Association of India, had pointed out that the health services in India "are in advance stage of decay" (ibid.).

As against WHO recommendation of 5 per cent, Central Government expenditure on public health has reduced from 1.3 per cent of gross domestic product (GDP) in 1990 to 0.9 per cent in 1999. Recently, there has been slight increase in budgetary allocation for health and it is expected that in the next five years, it will be increased up to 2-3 per cent of GDP (Shiva Kumar, 2005).

The increased 2005-06 budget allocation for Rajiv Gandhi National Drinking Water Mission from Rs 3,300 crore to Rs 4,700 crore and additional allocation of Rs 630 crore for sanitation to cover 452 districts of India (Shiva Kumar, ibid.) are definitely a positive step towards curbing the communicable diseases. However, the extent to which it will benefit the tribal population, is yet to be seen.

In view of dismal performances of PHCs in India, the increased access to modern medicines and health care is largely due to privatisation of health care. It has severe implications for the tribal population and economically poor sections of the society. For a community, which mainly survives on subsistence economy, its access to health care is increasingly being expensive. The privatised health care, being highly expensive, largely becomes inaccessible to these groups. They are, therefore, left with traditional system of medicines, superstition and magico-religious healing practices.

As a disadvantaged and marginalised group, the health situation of tribal population needs special attention. The tribes of India which are comparatively secluded, remotely situated, less educated, traditionally organised, materially impoverished and dispossessed, and economically exploited and underdeveloped, are one of the most vulnerable groups in India as is evident from the forthcoming discussions.

The sub-group on Rural Health and Indian Systems of Medicine and Homeopathy, constituted by the Planning Commission, Government of India and chaired by Alok Mukhopadhyay has recommended in its report that approximately one-third of the people of our country, particularly living in the tribal, hilly and arid as well as feudal areas have a critical health status. Their health problems are very much associated with the issues of food security and underdevelopment. The health of this population is directly linked to their economic, social and political status. It is quite clear from the findings of all social development ministries that there is a need to think of a sub-plan for the vulnerable and deprived regions. Major thrust should be to help them reverse the situation through a well planned, adequately financed community-oriented Integrated Health and Development Programmes with substantial participation from voluntary organisations.

Inequality, Poverty and Malnutrition

The wide gap between rich and poor is not only due to economic inequalities but also due to "inequality of opportunites". This dimension has assumed special significance in the context of economic reform, privatisation and globalisation. It is likely to further intensify the inequality by marginalising the poor and the tribal population because the expanded economic opportunities are difficult to be used if ill-health or illiteracy (Roy et al., 2004; Radhakrishna et al., 2004) handicaps a person. Education and health are two main influences, which promote the freedom and capability of individuals to make use of available opportunities (Dreze and Sen, 1995).

Data collected from a national sample of 35,000 rural household from 16 states by National Council of Applied Economic Research (NCAER), New Delhi in May 1994, suggests that increase in income leads to steady and systematic increase in literacy, considerable increase in enrolment, higher proportion of completing middle level of schooling and a fall in discontinuation rates (Shariff and Sudershan, 1996). It is evident that tribal communities being the poorest of the lot (Radhakrishna et al., 2004), remain far behind in terms of achievement of literacy, effecting thereby their capability to make use of available opportunities. It also has a limiting effect on their capability to improve their health through hygiene and awareness. NCAER (1994) data provides considerable differentials in levels of literacy among Scheduled Tribes as compared to other social categories (see Table 8.1).

The prevalence rate of morbidity is also found to be higher in economically weaker sections such as STs and SCs and wage

Table 8.1

Education Indicators by Social Groups in India

Social Groups	*Literacy Rate (7+ yrs.)*			*Net Enrolment rate (6-14 yrs.)*			*Discontinuation Rate (6-14 yrs.)*			*Proportion of Adult Population completing middle education*		
	F	*M*	*F/M*	*F*	*M*	*F/M*	*F*	*M*	*F/M*	*F*	*M*	*F/M*
STs	26	51	51	52	68	76	8	6.6	121	5.4	11.2	48
All	40	66	61	65	77	84	7.6	4.8	158	8.6	15.3	56

Source: Shariff and Sudershan (1996) – NCAER/HDI data 1994.

labourers. Taking into account the various causes of non- or under-reporting of morbidity, it looks as though the data available for tribal societies could be much higher as these factors are more prominent in these groups (ibid.) The NCAER data shows the considerably higher prevalence of diarrhea fever and T. B. among tribes of rural India as shown in Table 8.2.

Table 8.2

Short Duration Morbidity Prevalence Rate (MPR(SD)) and Major Morbidity Prevalence Rate (PPR(MM)) by Population Groups in Rural India

Social Groups	*Short Duration Morbidity: '000 Population*				*Major Illness per lac Population*	
	Diarrhea	*Cold/ Cough*	*Fever*	*MPR (SD)*	*T. B.*	*PPR (MM)*
STs						
Male	40	60	35	125	575	3566
Female	35	69	39	135	343	3117
Person	38	64	37	130	464	3377
All Groups						
Male	32	69	24	117	525	4571
Female	30	75	28	127	310	4585
Person	31	72	25	122	423	4578

Source: Shariff and Sudershan (1996).

In spite of free health care services in India, the household expenditure on treatment of sickness is large, i.e., Rs 273 per person annually; Rs 1,351 per household. It amounts to 5.3 per cent of average household income of Rs 25,653 (ibid.). Rich spend more in absolute term. With large and thriving private market in health care in India and the cuts on public expenditure on health in the context of structural adjustment, programmes are likely to adversely effect the vulnerable groups particularly the tribals (see Table 8.3).

Table 8.3

Expenditure on Treatment of Short Duration and Major Illness Per Person by Population Groups

Social Groups	*Annual Exp. on Short-term Illness (Rs.)*			*Annual Exp. on Long-term Illness (Rs.)*		
	Male	*Female*	*Person*	*Male*	*Female*	*Person*
ST	137	140	139	41	27	34
SC	1665	151	158	65	62	63
Other Hindus	169	160	1664	84	79	82
All groups	168	155	162	79	71	75

Source: Shariff and Sudershan (1996) – NCAER/HDI data 1994.

While a large number of primary health centres and sub-centres have been created as part of the government's Health for All programme, National Family Health Survey (NFHS) 1 and 2 reveal that health services either do not reach disadvantaged sections or are not accessed by them. The tribal population is adversely placed in terms of access to health care and nutritional status due to low economic condition, social hierarchy and stratification. Roy et al. (2004) have analysed the data from NFHS-2 conducted in 1998-99 on nationally representative sample of 92,486 households and 90,303 ever-married women age 15-49 in all 26 states that existed at the time of survey. In the country as a whole the deprivation and inequality of the tribal population in terms of eight indications as compared to other caste groups is the highest as revealed in Table 8.4:

Table 8.4

Percentage of Women with Selected Socioeconomic, Health and Nutritional Indicators by Caste and Tribe (NFHS-2, 1998-99)

Indicator	*STs*	*SCs*	*OBCs*	*Other*	*All*
Poverty/low standard of living	53.59	50.2	32.3	20.3	32.8
Illiterate	78.9	72.8	60.8	43.8	57.9
No media exposure	61.8	48.2	40.6	30.9	40.1
No health facilities within locality	58.1	42.4	40.3	31.2	38.7
No ANC	43.6	38.5	35.0	28.1	33.9
Unsafe Delivery	77.0	63.0	55.0	51.0	57.2
Low Body Mass Index (BMI $< 18.5 kg/m^3$)	46.6	42.6	36.2	30.8	36.1
Prevalence of any anaemia	64.9	56.0	50.7	47.7	51.8

Source: Roy et al., 2004.

The data shows that health status of tribal women is worst as compared to other social groups, which also indicates the risk of high malnutrition among tribes (Radhakrishna et al., 2004). It has been reported that there has been substantial reduction in poverty during 1970-2001 but alarmingly the rural urban gaps in performance of poverty reduction has widened. 1990s has witnessed the faster poverty reduction in urban areas due to the economic urban economic growth induced by privatisation and globalisation. It is also noteworthy that the percentage of poor in India is concentrated among SCs and STs which together accounts for 45 per cent of total poor persons in India which is much higher than their proportionate population. The incidence of poverty along with prevalence of very poor among tribes is the highest both in rural (44.2%, 22.1%) and urban areas (37.5%, 24.0%) as compared to other social groups. During the decade while the distribution of poor among other social categories have slightly reduced, among tribes it has increased from 14.8 per cent of total poor in 1993-94 to 17.5 per cent in 1999-00 (ibid.) as evident from the Table 8.5. It assumes significance with respect to increased reporting malnutrition related deaths of children largely from tribal areas (EPW, 2005).

Table 8.5

Percentage Distribution of Poor by Social Categories in Rural Areas

Category	*1993-94*	*1999-00*
SCs	27.6	27.3
STs	14.8	17.5
Others	57.6	55.2
All groups	100.0	100.0

Source: Radhakrishna et al., 2004.

It is noted also noted that deficiency of essential components in diet of tribal communities leading to malnutrition, protein calorie malnutrition and micro-nutrient deficiencies (vitamin A, iron and iodine) are common. Goitre of various grades is also endemic in some of the tribal areas particularly in Maharashtra. Water-borne and communicable diseases, i.e., gastrointestinal disorders particularly dysentery and parasitic infections are very common, leading to marked morbidity and malnutrition. Malaria and tuberculosis still remain a problem in many tribal areas (Kate, 2000).

Genetic and Endemic Diseases among Indian Tribes

There are some pressing problems of genetic disorder faced by Indian tribes such as sickle cell anaemia and Glucose-6 Phosphate Enzyme Deficiency (G-6-PD). Disease incidence for sickle-cell anaemia has been estimated at more than 19 per cent among 35 tribal population groups. About 5 million are estimated to be carriers of this disease (Basu, 1994).

Kate (2000) has studied the prevalence of sickle cell anaemia among tribe of Maharashtra. He suggests, on the basis of genetic survey data, that there is high prevalence of genetic disorders mostly involving red blood cells: Genetically transmitted disorders like sickle cell anaemia, G-6-PD and different forms of thalassaemia are also common. All these defects lead to the early destruction of red blood cells and add to the overall anaemia. Sickle cell disorder in the overall population of Maharashtra is less than 0.1 per cent while it is very high amongst the tribal population groups, i.e., tribes like Oktar, Pardhan, Pawara, Media, Gond and Bhil having more than 20 per cent carriers. Some of the common symptoms seen in patients suffering from sickle cell anaemia include – anaemia, intermittent jaundice, severe joint pains and recurrent infections. These symptoms usually appear between the ages of four and five and severity increases with age. In the absence of any cure, majority of the sickle cell patients have a miserable and a short lifespan.

G-6-PD shows a genetically carried deficiency in a blood enzyme; persons commonly reject antimalarials, antibiotics, and analgesics. The population estimated to have the deficiency is about 13 million, primarily residing in Madhya Pradesh, Maharashtra, Tamil Nadu, Orissa, and Assam states (15%). The incidence is high in malaria zones (Basu, 1994).

The Onges, Jarawas, and Shompens of Andaman and Nicobar Islands are facing extinction due to endemic diseases (Basu, 1994). There is alarmingly high prevalence rate of Hepatitis B infection has been detected among the tribal people of the Andaman and Nicobar Islands. Compared to the average 4 to 5 per cent rate in the general population of mainland India, the prevalence rate in these tribal populations is over 20 per cent, the highest recorded in recent times. Epidemiologically, more that 8 per cent prevalence is termed as "high endemicity". A majority of Hepatitis B carriers are asymptomatic. The infection is self-limiting but in chronic carriers of the virus, it ultimately affects the liver leading to cirrhosis, cancer and other serious manifestations of the liver. It is for this reason the infection is termed as a silent killer (Ramchandran, 2000).

Antenatal Care and Knowledge about AIDS

Due to the lack of curative and preventive medicines the awareness and knowledge about AIDS is the only appropriate strategy for its control and spread prevention. India has the highest number of HIV infected people in the world with 3.9 million infection which spread very fast during 1990s from high risk population to general population through occupation and migration (Sambamoorthi et al., 2004). The estimate shows that by 2001, women in India accounted for 25 per cent of case load and 90 per cent of the infections were found to be occurring in persons under 50 years of age, the chances of epidemic spread through child-bearing women to the children has become higher (ibid.). Due to impoverishment and unemployment, a significant number of tribal labourers migrates to nearby towns and cities. Thus the so-called secluded tribal communities are exposed and made even more vulnerable to this epidemic. Micro studies suggest that many Indians lack the adequate knowledge about AIDS. A study in Delhi showed that 56 per cent of the sample had not even heard of the disease (ibid.). On the basis of National Family Health Survey 1998-99 (NFHS-2) data, Sambamoorthi et al., have calculated that only 46.9 per cent of ever married tribal women aged between 18 and 48 years with at least one birth in the past three years prior to the study, ever had antenatal care. It was found to be the lowest as compared to other social categories, i.e., SC (56.2%), Backward (59.5%) and Other (68.8%). Majority (53.1%) of tribal women of the national sample never had antenatal care.

It is important to note that pre-natal care is important to reduce the risk of transmission of HIV. The study also finds that only 35.5 per cent of women of all categories had any awareness about AIDS, which is alarmingly very low in itself; the rate of AIDS awareness was all the more lowest among the tribal women, ie., 17 per cent (ibid.). The result shows that tribal groups are highly susceptible and vulnerable to the spread of HIV infection as far as AIDS awareness is concerned.

The Mungana Experience

The findings of Mungana Survey (Prayas, 2005) provide very useful micro-level feel of the tribal health scenario and interestingly supports the severity of tribal health status as compared to most of the issues discussed above, except the genetic and endemic disease issue, since this dimension was not probed during the survey. The southern part of Rajasthan accounts for highest concentration of its tribal population. The data provided by 'Prayas' is based on a pilot survey conducted on 2,275 individuals of 405 randomly selected tribal families within 10 villages of 'Mungana' Panchayat of Dhariawad tehsil in Udaipur district. Most of the families surveyed are related to Bhil tribe, which predominantly inhabits this part of Rajasthan.

The economic condition of these families is very poor. Though income of the family was not directly asked but it is evident from the fact that almost all the families residing in 'kachcha' houses, 402 or 99.3 per cent engage in subsistence agriculture as their primary occupation and 86.4 per cent families had to supplement their incomes by working as labourers. Only 2 families were found in service. Curiously enough, only 19 per cent (77 families) were included in the BPL listing of the Government and hold the Red Card. Out of these only 47 (11.6%) had the health card.

Hygienic condition can be estimated to be very poor through two indicators, i.e., source of drinking water and post relieving hand wash methods. Around 52.8 per cent population drinks water from the hand-pump, rest of the population uses open well or the natural stream. Thus, almost half of the population uses unsafe drinking water. It is also an area which is known for the attack of thread worm (Nadu disease in the local dialect). Due to awareness and lot of government propaganda people have started using the water after filtering it through the cloth and the occurrence of the disease has nearly vanished in recent decade.[2] But the use of water from open well and stream still remains open to all kind of microbial contamination. As is the general patterns in the rural areas, most of the people go to open fields for relieving themselves; it was found that 98 per cent of them use soil to wash their hands and even less than 2 per cent only use ash or soap for the purpose.

Population related figures show that the average family size was 5.9. The sex ratio is fastly declining. While it was found to be 1010 among the adult population (above 15 years of age); it had dropped by 88 points to be 922 among the younger population (below 15 years' group). Early marriage is a common practice among these people and as a result one-third of the women had delivered their first baby when below 17 years of age. Literacy rates are low too as compared to the national averages. While the general literacy rate is 51 per cent; among women it is 44 per cent and among men it is 57 per cent.

Looking at the state of immunisation of children, we find that there are 435 children between the age-group of 0-5 years. Out of these, 175 (40.2%) have been given the BCG vaccine; and only 10(2.2%) have received the khasra vaccine. Though 68 (15.63%) have taken the first DPT vaccine, out of these, only 27 (39.70%) and 19 (27.94%) have taken the second and the third dose of DPT respectively. Therefore, only 4.36 per cent are immunised against DPT. Similar is the case with polio, where only 35 (8.04%) who have taken the first polio vaccine and the number has decreased to 20 (57.14%) at the second and 13 (37.14%) at the third level of polio immunisation. Thus, only 2.98 per cent are immunised against polio.

Women's health is a prime concern nationwide. In Mungana, an average of four deliveries per woman was calculated. While the number of women was 511, the number of deliveries was 2,110. This figure includes abortions. Out of these, only 421 (20%) have taken the tetanus vaccine, 300 (14%) have taken the iron tablets and 29 and 23 women (2.4%) had got the urine and the blood tests done respectively. If we exclude the abortions, then out of total 2,059 deliveries, 1,795 (87.18%) were done by untrained Dais and 264 (12.82%) were done by a nurse or a doctor. About 1,799 (87.37%) were done at home and 261 (12.67%) were done at the hospital. Out of those done at home, maternity kit (Mamta) was used in 219 cases and the rest were unsafe births. Thus, we see that 61 (3% approx.) still-born babies were delivered and 189 babies (9.18%) died between the age of 0-1 years. The Child Mortality rate for the sample was calculated to be 5 per cent.

Family planning figures show that only 7.5 per cent people have planned their family and 13.5 per cent are willing to take one or the other family planning measure. Out of 796 married people, two had used Copper T and 4 intended to use it, one had used Mala-D and 31 were willing to use it. Around five women had used local herbs and one intended to use it in the future; and while 52 women had undergone sterilisation, 72 were intending to do the same.

Thus, the tribal health situation in these villages is characterised by very little pre- and post-natal maternal care. It has high incidence of unsafe births under almost nil trained medical supervision, high mortality rate, very low level of child immunisation, early girl child marriage with declining sex ratio in younger population, poor hygienic standards and use of unsafe drinking water coupled with poverty and low level of literacy.

Voluntary Sector and Tribal Health

In spite of good policies and positive intentions, the direct intervention of government health machinery in tribal areas is barest to the minimum. The void generated is to some extent being filled by the voluntary efforts. It is needless to say that these efforts are largely haphazard, eclectic and fund driven. Their concerns are dominated by the priorities of the funding agencies and they often lack proper probing of local health issues preceding their intervention, neither do these come under any macro and long-term nationwide health perspective relating to the tribal communities.

Due to the difficulty in approaching the remote and secluded tribal settlements, utter neglect of government health officials and the distant availability of primary health care to these communities are well known bottle-necks in improving the health status of these groups. In this regard the voluntary sector should be strategically involved in providing primary health care in a more effective manner, in these areas. As suggested by sub-group on Rural health and Indian Systems of Medicine and Homeopathy, constituted by the Planning Commission, Government of India, and chaired by Alok Mukhopadhayay, special fund like Council for Advancement of People's Action and Rural Technology (CAPART) should be set aside for this purpose. It should also play an important role in imparting health education through schools and other fora. The services of qualified voluntary organisations should be utilised for training of community health workers as well as for giving continuing education to other health personnel of the government. Similarly, they should be partners in the programme of eradication of TB and malaria throughout the country. Given the growing professional competency of the voluntary organisations and some successful experiments on various aspects of health care, they should be involved in the process of planning and monitoring of health services both at the central as well as at state levels.

The Way Forward: Miles To Go!

The tribal population is a very important segment of our society and culture. In a situation when some of the Indian tribes are on the verge of extinction and rest due to impoverishment, illiteracy and seclusion become the most vulnerable group of our society. Their health needs are not only unique because they have peculiar health problems such as genetic disorder and endemic diseases in some pockets but also for common health problems they happen to be the most vulnerable group. With growing privatisation of health services along with growing incidence of poverty among them, their health needs demand special and immediate attention. It a daunting task for the government and civil society as well. It demands an integrated approach to improve their economic, educational and health conditions.

In order to improve the health situation of tribal population following steps are urgent need of the time:

- Formulation of sub-plan for vulnerable population and deprived region with special attention to the needs of tribal population.
- Improvement of health infrastructure and functioning of PHC in tribal areas.
- Training the local medical practitioners, doctors of non-allopathic systems, traditional healers and Dayees from the tribal community to deal with the local common health needs.
- Involvement of local community/panchayat in health administration and awareness generation.
- Ensuring the improvement of nutritional level particularly of mother and children.
- Ensuring complete immunisation of their children.
- Proper training to the PHC medical staff to detect the presence of common genetic disorders and to mark them with tattoo.

- Ensuring the curb on health hazards caused by developmental projects in tribal areas.
- Carry out population genetic survey programme to detect carriers and suffers.
- Imparting health education and awareness regarding common as well as genetic disorder.
- Provide genetic counselling and follow-up genetically disordered persons.

(We duly acknowledge the generosity of Prayas, Chittorgarh – Dr. Narendra Gupta and Miss Anjali in particular – for sharing Munagana pilot survey findings with us. It has proven to be the valuable input for this paper. Our gratitude also to the motivation, encouragement, library support and feed-backs provided by Satyapal B. Seth, New Delhi without which this effort could never have materialised.)

Notes

1. Prayas is a voluntary organisation working in Chittorgarh and adjacent areas of Udaipur district of South Rajasthan. Major constituent of target communities of 'Prayas' is tribal and improvement of health status is one of its core concern.
2. We came to know about the prevalence and eradication of this disease from Prof. Yogendra Singh during a discussion in Delhi a few years back.

References

Basu, S.K. (1993): 'Health Status of Tribal Women in India', *Social Change*, December 1993, 23(4), pp. 19-39. http://www.hsph.harvard.edu/Organizations/healthnet/SAsia/forums/Tribals/Tribals/M002.HTM.

Basu, S.K. (1994): 'A Health Profile of Tribal India', *Health for Millions*, April 2 (2):12-4.

Banerji, Debabar (2005): 'Politics of Rural Health in India', *Economic and Political Weekly*, Vol. 40 No. 30, July 23-29:3253-58.

Dreze, J. and A. Sen (1995): *India Economic Development and Social Opportunity*, OUP, Delhi.

Economic and Political Weekly (2005): 'Child Malnutrition' Vol. 40 No. 36, September 3-9:3380.

Kate S.L. (2000): 'Health Problems of Tribal Population Groups from the State of Maharashtra', *Immunohaematology Bulletin*, October 23, http://mail.yahoo.com/config/login?/_javascript:openWin (india_tribes.html).

Phadke, Anant (2003): 'Right to Health Care', *Economic and Political Weekly*, Vol. 38 No. 41, Oct. 11-17:4308-09.

Prayas (2005): Pilot Survey Report – Mungana (Dhariyawad). Chittorgarh (unpublished).

Radhakrishna R., K. Hanumantha Rao, C. Ravi and B. Sammi Reddy (2004): 'Chronic Poverty and Malnutrition in 1990s', *Economic and Political Weekly* Vol. 39 No. 28, July 10-16: 3121-30.

Ramchandran, R. (2000): 'A People in Peril', *Frontline* Vol. 17 – Issue 16, August 5-18: http://www.flonnet.com/

Roy, T.K., S. Kulkarni and Y. Vaidehi (2004): 'Social Inequalities in Health and Nutrition in Selected States', *Economic and Political Weekly* Vol. 39 No. 7, Feb.14-20:667-683.

Sambamoorthi Usha, Rakkee Thimothy, Wenhui Wei and S Irudaya Rajan (2004): 'Antenatal Care and AIDS: Knowledge Among Married Women', *Economic and Political Weekly* Vol. 39 No. 7, Feb 14-20:721-27.

Sarin, Madhu (2005): 'Scheduled Tribes Bill 2005 – A Comment', *Economic and Political Weekly* Vol. 40 No. 21, May 21-27: 2121-34.

Shariff, Abusaleh and Ratna M. Sudarshan (1996): 'Elementary Education and Health in Rural India: Some indicators' in Rao N., L. Rurup and R Sudarshan (ed.) *Site of Change*, FES and UNDP, New Delhi: 45-117.

Shiva Kumar, A.K. (2005): 'Budgeting for Health', *Economic and Political Weekly*, Vol. 40 No. 14, April 2-8.

9

Sexually Transmitted Diseases among the Tribal Women of Reproductive Span

Chakrapani Upadhyay

Sexuality tends to be evaluated according to categories of natural/unnatural, normal/abnormal, and moral/immoral sexual behaviour. These terms are value judgements, reflecting social norms rather than any quality inherent in the behaviour itself (Nataraja, 1995). Human sexuality is characterised by sexual variation from "never" to "always", from "normal" to "deviant". The culture, caste, community and socio-economic class exert an influence on sexual behaviour. Popular culture both encourages and discourages sexuality. It promotes stereotypical sexual interactions between men and women that fail to touch on the deeper significance sexuality holds for us. Marital love and sexuality are infrequently depicted in contrast to casual or non-marital sex (Turner, 1996). The variety of sexual behaviours testifies to diversity not only between cultures but within cultures as well. Understanding diversity allows us to acknowledge that there is no such thing as inherently "normal" or "natural" sexual behaviour.

Certain population groups are more at risk than others to contact sexually transmitted diseases (STDs). These groups include people under-25, minorities, the medically undeserved and gay men the African-Americans, the urban low-income group, etc. (Turner, 1996). In India the tribal groups are covered in this category. A number of reasons explain their vulnerability: inadequate medical services, higher rates of other diseases, unsanitary living conditions, overcrowding, ignorance about STDs. Traditional health system, language and culture are also barriers to the treatment of STDs.

A sexually transmitted disease (STD) is a contagious infection that, for the most part, is passed on by intimate sexual contact with others. It is an umbrella term for various infections transmitted by sexual contact, including chancroid, chlamydia, genital herpes, and gonorrhoea, human papillomavirus, syphilis, and trichomoniasis.

Sexually transmitted disease embodies a kind of biological sexism but its spread through cultural setting of society depends on the degree of permissiveness. Frequently men have no complaints or clinical symptoms in the early phases of the disease (particularly gonorrhoea and syphilis) and therefore fail to get treatment. They also suffer more serious long-term consequences from all STDs (ibid.). Moreover, women are more likely than men to contact an STD from any single sexual encounter and suffer more than double the disease burden than men (Panthaki, 1998). The limited studies available on this subject generally paint a grim picture of high morbidity and malnutrition among Indian girls and women (Bhatia and Cleland, 1995; Chatterjee, 1991; Chidambaram, Soorasangaran and Anbuganapathi, 1986; Rao, Marwah, Tiwari, Murthy, Gupta and Dwive, 1973). A new problem that is spreading rapidly is HIV/AIDS, which will significantly affect the health of Indian women.

Among the sexually transmitted diseases, Acquired Immuno-Deficiency Syndrome (AIDS) is a condition characterised by a breakdown of the body's immune system that makes people vulnerable to a variety of infections, certain forms of cancer, and various neurological disorders. AIDS is caused by a virus named Human Immuno-deficiency Virus (HIV), which lives and reproduces inside human cells and is transmitted by blood and blood products (such as plasma), semen, vaginal secretions, and possibly breast milk (Turner, 1996; Delaney, 1992). Because there is no cure, AIDS is a fatal condition, although patients are now surviving longer than they did just a few years ago, thanks to new medical treatments (Brayn, 1994). What distinguishes AIDS from many other fatal diseases is that it is preventable (Centres for Disease Control and Prevention, 1993).

AIDS is a collection of diseases caused by the Human Immuno-Deficiency Virus (HIV). The disorder is characterised by a specific defect in the body's immune system. The WHO estimates 6,000 new infections of HIV daily. The exigencies of AIDS prevention necessarily create tensions between the need to lessen women subordination on the one hand and the need to prevent women from infection on a daily basis on the other (Turner, 1996).

Social Factors of STDs and AIDS

STDs and AIDS do not represent solely a medical problem. They are symptoms of a wider social pathology in the community (Park, 1986). The social factors implicated in the spread of STDs and AIDS may be summarised as follows:

(a) *Prostitution:* The common denominator in the spread of STDs and AIDS is prostitution. The prostitute acts as a reservoir of infection. The male supplies a demand: if there were no prostituants, there would be no prostitutes.

(b) *Broken homes:* Social studies indicate that promiscuous women usually come from broken homes, where the atmosphere is unhappy. Children reared therein are likely to go astray in search of other avenues of happiness.

(c) *Easy money:* Prostitution provides an occupation for earning easy money.

(d) *Emotional immaturity:* The incidence of STDs and AIDS in the age group 15-19 years is very high, especially in girls This has been attributed to emotional immaturity.

(g) *Urbanisation and industrialisation:* These have led to an extensive floating population in cities, towns, ports, and industrial areas and a greater opportunity for sexual encounter.

(h) *Population mobility:* Increased population movement by air, land and sea (e.g., tourists, migrant workers) – an important factor in the spread of STDs and AIDS.

(i) *Greater sexual encounter:* More female employment, co-educational schooling and college learning cause greater opportunities for sexual encounter.

(j) *Changing behavioural patterns:* Greater tolerance in sexual behaviour, frequent pre-marital and extramartial intercourse, sexual freedom and community living are changing behavioural patterns.

(k) *Population increase:* Implies higher student population and more young people at risk.

(l) *Economic factors*: Rapid economic development. Greater prosperity and affluence allows people greater freedom to get away and enjoy sex.

(m) *Homosexuality:* Great deal of male STD infection is reported to be homosexually transmitted. Homosexual men have much higher rates of gonorrhoea and syphilis than heterosexual men.

(n) *Chastity:* Chastity is a safeguard against STDs and AIDS. In modern society the value traditionally set upon chastity is in conflict with the more recent ideas of independence and freedom from supervision and equal rights for both sexes. There has been a relaxation of moral and cultural values in present-day society. The tendency to break away from traditional ways of life is particularly marked among young people.

(o) *Social stigma:* Social stigma is attached to STDs and AIDS. This factor leads to shyness, which accounts for the non-detection of cases. The patient does not avail medical services, does not disclose the source of contact, gives a wrong address to avoid identification, goes to quacks for treatment and drops out before the treatment is complete.

(p) *Contraceptives:* The new methods of contraception and liberalisation of abortion laws have reduced the fear of illness and pregnancy.

(q) *Self-treatment:* In many countries penicillin and other drugs are easily available without a prescription. As a result many infected persons treat themselves. This has resulted in an attitude of indifference to the dangers of the STDs and AIDS. A large number of "repeaters" belong to this group.

(r) *Alcoholism:* The associations of alcohol and STDs and AIDS have often been noted. Alcoholism and prostitution mutually cause the damage done to their consumers.

(s) *Local marriage customs:* The high incidence of STDs and AIDS in some areas may be associated with the local marriage customs of polyandry and polygamy.

Objectives and Methodology

The main objectives of the present study are:

1. Analyse the social factors related to STDs and AIDS among the tribes,
2. Correlate the socio-demographic characteristics of the tribes with their sexually transmitted diseases,

3. Assess the awareness about HIV/AIDS, STDs, sexually transmitted infection (STI) and reproductive tract infection (RTI) in tribal society,
4. Analyse the socio-cultural factors among the tribes with reference to STDs and AIDS epidemic.
5. Analyse the determinants of sexually transmitted diseases with their contribution to the problem.

Magnitude of the problems of STDs increases because of the following reasons:

- Sexual initiation occurs relatively early, by ages 17-19 years in most cases (Goparaju, 1993).
- Adolescents are poorly informed about their own sexuality and physical well-being. Whatever knowledge they have is incomplete and confusing.
- Awareness of sexually transmitted disease and AIDS is 25 per cent and 32 per cent amongst poorer and younger adolescent girls and boys respectively (Bhende,1995).
- According to WHO, at least half of those infected with HIV are under 25, with the 15-19 age group having the second highest rates of AIDS.

Looking at the nature and objectives of the study, it was considered appropriate to use exploratory, descriptive and comparative research design. The WHO recommended 30 cluster sampling technique was used to obtain the requisite information from 300 women respondents. Two participatory focus group discussions (FGD) were conducted in the study area. For the present study, the information about socio-cultural and demographic determinants were collected by the individual interview of the mothers who have experienced at least one delivery in the last five years with the help of a structured interview schedule. In regression analysis two sets of variables are used namely, independent and dependent indicators. Total nine dependants and thirteen independent indicators are computed for stepwise regression equation. To access the determinants some indicators are made. The present study was conducted in Dungarpur district. It reveals how the position of tribal Bhil and Meena women affects their sexual health.

Myths and Misconceptions Related to STDs and HIV/AIDS

Several reasons have been mentioned about myths and misconceptions of sexually transmitted diseases. Generally observed among them are as follows:

- Most sexually transmitted diseases are the product of modern times.
- STD is a punishment for immoral or promiscuous behaviour.
- STD and HIV can be contacted by contact with a toilet seat or by using a public toilet.
- A person can catch STD from using some eating utensils.
- Washing one's private part's everyday is sufficient to prevent a STD.
- Birth control pills protect you from STDs.
- If one has syphilis or gonorrhoea one will know it.
- STD infections in the genitals cannot be transmitted to the mouth, and vice versa.
- If a man with a sexually transmitted disease has sex with a virgin girl he will be cured of STD.
- Disappearance of the symptoms implies cure of the STD.
- Once you have been cured of a STD, you cannot get it again.

Myths and misconceptions about HIV/AIDS are as under:

- HIV was developed in the laboratory as germ warfare against gay or blacks. It was spread through contaminated vaccines.
- If you are HIV-positive, it means you have AIDS.
- The AIDS virus is easy to "catch".
- HIV is spread through household pets and from animals.

- HIV is transmitted by the bite of insects such as mosquitoes.
- HIV is live and replicates in water. It is transmitted in drinking water, tubs or swimming pools.
- HIV can be spread through everyday social contacts, such as touching or being near a person with AIDS.
- HIV is found in the sweat and tears of HIV-infected people.
- A person carrying HIV cannot pass it on to others unless that person has developed AIDS symptoms.
- Women cannot transmit HIV to their sex partners.
- Latex condoms have naturally acquiring holes that are sometimes bigger than HIV so condoms do not really provide protection against the HIV.
- HIV does not cause AIDS.
- You can have AIDS without HIV.
- HIV is extremely difficult to kill on surfaces.
- It is HIV itself that eventually kills the person.
- If you are not in high-risk group you do not have to worry about AIDS. In other words, "low risk means no risk."
- Scientists have not actually seen an AIDS virus.
- AIDS is a disease of homosexuals.
- AIDS will take care of the problem of over population explosion.

Awareness about HIV/AIDS, STDs, STIs and RTIs

Awareness of HIV and AIDS, sexually transmitted diseases (STDs) and reproductive tract infections (RTIs) among the tribal women are analysed with reference to the background characteristics. The findings are reported in Table 9.1. About 80 per cent women are aware of HIV and AIDS. The awareness is very high in urban areas (94%). As the age increases the level of awareness decreases; there is a negative correlation between the current age and awareness about HIV/AIDS. Eleven women in every dozen, aged between 20-24 years, know about HIV.

No significant HIV awareness-related differences are found among both the Bhil and Meena tribes.

Table 9.1

Awareness about HIV/AIDS, STD, STI and RTI Percentage Distribution of Women by Selected Background Characteristics, According to Awareness about HIV/AIDS, STDs, STIs and RTIs

Characteristics	*Awareness about*				*Number*
	HIV/AIDS	*STD*	*STIs*	*RTIs*	
Residence					
Rural	74.20	18.30	10.90	11.40	229
Urban	94.20	25.00	22.50	19.70	71
Current Age					
15-19	100.00	0.00	0.00	0.00	24
20-24	92.60	23.50	17.60	13.20	68
25-29	86.60	27.30	31.80	36.40	44
30-34	74.20	24.20	15.20	13.60	66
35-39	51.30	25.60	7.70	10.30	39
40-44	89.70	17.20	6.90	6.90	29
45-49	53.30	3.30	0.00	0.00	30
Tribe					
Bhil	79.10	20.20	14.00	15.50	129
Meena	78.90	19.90	13.50	11.70	171
Religion					
Hindu	78.30	20.60	14.20	13.50	281
Christian	66.70	16.70	16.70	16.70	6
Not stated	100.00	7.70	0.00	7.70	13
Family					
Nuclear	76.50	20.20	12.60	11.30	238
Joint	88.70	19.40	17.70	21.00	62
House					
Kachcha	74.20	17.20	11.30	11.10	221
Pucca	96.30	33.30	22.20	19.20	27
Semi-Pucca	90.40	25.00	19.20	12.20	52

Contd...

Contd...

Education					
Illiterate	74.90	16.30	7.00	8.40	227
Literate	90.00	25.00	25.00	15.00	20
Primary	92.00	24.00	20.00	24.00	25
Middle	100.00	25.40	30.80	27.70	13
Secondary	90.90	81.80	81.80	72.70	11
Sr. Secondary	75.00	25.00	50.00	75.00	4
Husband's Education					
Illiterate	71.00	16.60	7.10	10.10	169
Literate	77.30	18.20	9.10	13.60	22
Primary	92.80	16.00	10.00	8.00	50
Middle	85.00	30.00	60.00	20.00	20
Secondary	100.00	30.00	35.00	25.00	20
Sr. Secondary	83.30	41.70	50.00	25.00	12
Graduate and above	100.00	42.90	42.90	57.10	7
Occupation					
Housewife	84.40	26.70	20.70	19.30	136
Agriculture	65.00	1.30	1.30	1.30	80
Service	84.60	30.00	20.00	30.80	13
Labour	84.50	32.40	16.90	18.30	71
Husband's Occupation					
Unemployed	20.00	20.00	10.00	10.00	5
Domestic work	83.30	0.00	16.70	0.00	6
Agriculture	53.20	1.30	2.60	0.00	44
Service	95.30	25.90	20.00	20.00	85
Labour	81.00	29.10	1.10	13.90	79
Other	95.80	29.20	13.30	25.00	48
Total	79.00	20.00	13.70	13.30	300

Note: For Chi-square, please see Table 9.2.

Awareness about HIV is higher in women of joint families and those inhabiting *pakka* houses. As the level of education of the woman and for her husband increases, the awareness also increases. Two-thirds of the women engaged in agricultural activity know about HIV/AIDS. In service class about 90 per cent are aware about it. The awareness varies with change in husband's occupation also in a similar fashion.

Sexually transmitted diseases (STDs) have a direct relationship with reproductive health. The awareness about STDs is lesser than that about HIV/AIDS although the percentage tribals suffering from this affection is higher. One-fourth of the urban women and one-fifth of the rural women know about STDs. Women in cities have a greater access to modern therapeutic methods and more exposure to the media. Young tribal women are little aware about STD. Women aged between 45-49 years are also mostly unaware of the health risks passed by STDs. About one quarter of women of all the other age brackets affirmed awareness about STDs. Tribe-wise, Bhils have slightly better awareness than Meenas.

About one in every five women hailing from either nuclear or joint family background displayed awareness about STDs. The percentage of well-informed women inhabiting *pakka* houses is twice than those from *kacha* houses. Female education is a key indicator of awareness. In matriculated women awareness is five times greater than among illiterates. A similar trend is noted in the case of husband's education too. Occupation-wise, service class women are quite aware, housewives less so, while those pursuing agricultural activities are hardly aware about it. The husband's occupation and awareness about STDs follows a parallel pattern.

Sexually transmitted infections (STIs) may lead to STDs but the awareness about them is very low in tribal areas. The basic etiology of STI is the widespread promiscuity and the prevalence of socio-cultural practices like pre-marital and extra-marital sex.

Rural women display double the percentage of ignorance than urban women, very young and middle-aged women exhibit a lower level of awareness. The same holds for women from nuclear family set-up and *kacha* houses. Women educated up to secondary are highly aware about STIs (82%) in comparison with illiterate women (7%). As the educational level of the couple improves, the awareness level of the wife also increases. Women and men belonging to higher occupational strata show better realisation of the potential hazard of STI.

Reproductive tract infections (RTIs) are generally a result of the unhygienic measures undertaken and the consequent complication during pregnancy, delivery and post-partum period. Various socio-cultural beliefs, which govern the behaviour of tribal women, have a greater effect in rural areas than the urban. Women of the age group 20-24; 25-30 and 30-34 years are much more aware of RTIs than those are in the lower and higher age groups. Bhils are more aware than Meena tribal women. About one-fifth of the women of *pakka* houses and joint family set-up have a perception of the health problems associated with RTI. In a nuclear family set-up and *kacha* houses the awareness is almost half.

As the educational level of the women increases, the realisation about RTI maladies also follows. The husband's education also confirms greater level of awareness. The inference is that education and health-risk awareness are positively correlated.

Socio-cultural Factors of STDs and HIV/AIDS

Table 9.2 presents association of seven socio-cultural variables covering awareness about HIV/AIDS, STDs, RTIs and STIs problems, with selected socio-cultural factors.

Awareness about HIV/AIDS is widespread in tribal areas. Religion and type of tribe do not show any significant association with the awareness about these diseases. All other background characteristics are associated with awareness about HIV/AIDS at 0.01 level of significance. Awareness about sexually transmitted diseases is based on socio-educational and

Table 9.2

Socio-cultural Factors of STDs

Chi-Square,degree of freedom and level of significance by selected background characteristics of currently married women aged 15-49 years according to variables of STDs

	Awareness											
	HIV/AIDS			*STDs*			*RTIs*			*STIs*		
Characteristics	P2	*(df)*	*Sig*	P2	*(df)*	*Sig*	P2	*(df)*	*Sig*	P2	*(df)*	*Sig*
Residence	13.23	(01)	**	1.66	(01)		6.20	(01)	**	3.28	(01)	
Current Age	49.33	(06)	**	14.84	(06)	*	24.17	(06)	**	29.86	(06)	**
Tribe	0.006	(01)		0.003	(01)		0.01	(01)		0.92	(01)	
Religion	4.09	(02)		1.34	(02)		2.018	(02)		0.42	(02)	
Family	4.44	(01)	*	0.02	(01)		1.10	(01)		3.94	(01)	*
House	63.83	(02)	**	0.36	(02)		2.71	(02)		1.48	(02)	
Education	23.16	(05)	**	28.93	(05)	**	52.50	(05)	**	49.32	(05)	**
Husband's Education	35.46	(06)	**	15.49	(06)	**	35.12	(06)	**	26.55	(06)	*
Occupation	17.17	(04)	**	31.64	(04)	**	19.02	(04)	**	17.88	(04)	**
Husband's Occupation	71.65	(05)	**	28.04	(05)	**	26.76	(05)	**	22.48	(05)	**

Note: ** Chi-Square is significant at the 0.01 level.
* Chi-Square is significant at the 0.05 level.

socio-occupational status of the couple. Rural-urban, age, education and occupation show great differences in the level of awareness. Those having lower education and engaged in lower occupation are less aware about STDs. Similar trend is observed in associations about reproductive tract infections (RTIs) and sexually transmitted infections (STIs).

Behavioural Aspects of STDs

The term "behaviour" is often used in a socio-psychological perspective. It broadly covers various interactional aspects of individuals and their personality. An attempt has been made to study behavioural differentials of Bhil and Meenas. Sexual behaviour is a complex phenomenon with multiple dimensions. It is affected by cultural preferences of diverse roots and strengths and community feelings.

A behavioural differential (BD) scale was constructed to rate the differential responses of the women of reproductive age (15-49 years) and was used for all 300 respondents. The basis for the scale is rooted in the semantic differential propounded by Osgood (1957). In the study of health and sexual behaviour, this technique is considered useful in measuring the impact of cultural norms and traditions, beliefs and practices on women belonging to various categories. This is because it is a semi-projective technique and hence better than routine questionnaire or schedule method.

For framing of the BD scale 123 statements were selected on the basis of a pilot study. After assessing the variability, 98 such statements were formed to get a complete view. Six judges (sociologists, NGO workers and doctors of Preventive and Social Medicine) were asked to rate the appropriateness of each scale item on a five-point Likert type scale. The opinion of the judges was analysed and the statements, which were considered more appropriate by the judges, were included in the first format of sexual behavioural differential scale (SBDS).

There were 18 items in the first format of SBDS; it was pre-tested on 30 respondents. The responses were analysed and fourteen items were selected for the scale. The judges were shown these items, who suggested dropping four items. The final scale consisted of 10 items of sexual behaviour. Test-retest reliability was calculated after getting the responses of the same thirty persons included in the pre-tested sample. The reliability was found to be quite high (0.82). The small variation in response can be attributed to the different situational factors.

Dimensions of sexual behaviour have been identified using Component Method of Factor Analysis. The factor analyses shows five factors, out of which three factors, which account for greater degree of variance and which would be logically interpreted, are explained.

Factor 1: Sins

Disease, epidemics, sexual infection and illness is very common in tribal areas. Tribal women believe that various diseases are a result of their sins of previous births. They should take holy dip for cure of such diseases. This is taken in the river at Baneshwar Dham for good health. These beliefs are influenced by the household size, thus upheld by large families or joint families.

Factor 2: Malevolent Spirits

Tribal women have excessive faith in evil spirits, *Jadu-tona, Jhad-phoonk, Jantra-mantra* and amulets, etc. They believe that evil spirits are responsible for all diseases.. These evil spirits cause most of the sexual diseases and they invisibly have intercourse with women. The women go for Jhad-phoonk and the Ojha exhorts evil spirits out of their body. They tie amulets so that the spirits do not trouble them again. It is believed that evil spirits are afraid of these amulets.

Factor 3: Age

The third dimension of STDs is related to the couple's age. Belief about infection of sex organ and sexual disease is affected by age of the couple. If the couple is young they choose modern medical treatment, whereas elderly couples believe in Jhad-phoonk and Tona-totka. Aged women are likely to suffer more from diseases than the younger ones.

Table 9.3

Factor Analysis of STD Behavioural Differential Items

(N=300)

Factor No.	*Name*	*Items*	*Variable Name*	*Factor Loadings*
1	Sins	Illness is result of sins of earlier births	Sins	0.576
		For keeping health, go for holy dip	Holy dip	0.411
		Household size	Household size	0.402
2	Malevolent spirits	Get Jhad-Phoonk	Jhad-Phoonk	0.855
		Cured by tying amulets	Amulets	0.796
		Evil spirits cause diseases	Evil spirits	0.702
3	Age	Husband's current age	Husband's age	0.963
		Woman's current age	Woman's age	0.962

Extraction Method: Principal Component Analysis.

Rotation Method: Varimax with Kaiser Normalisation.

SPSS output

Determinants of Awareness about Sexually Transmitted Diseases

Two types of variables are used in the regression analysis, namely dependent and independent variables. The independent variables are the ones, which contribute in making the dependent variable. Several variables have been computed with the help of statements pertaining to sexual behaviour of the tribal women. The indicators used in the present study are made by combining relevant variables.

Table 9.4

Regression Determinants of Awareness About STD Among Tribal Women

	Dependent Variables: Awareness About STD		
Independent Variables	*Beta*	*Simple r*	*t-value*
Number of children ever born (CEB)	-0.28**	-0.28**	5.18
Husband's education	0.20**	0.27**	3.55
Residence	-0.11*	-0.18**	2.05

Multiple = 0.28

R Square = 0.08

* Significant at 0.05 level

** Significant at 0.01 level

SPSS output

Table 9.4 reveals that awareness about sexually transmitted diseases (STDs) can be predicted by three independent variables namely number of children ever born (CEB), husband's education and residence. The combined contribution of these three variable is eight per cent ($R^2 = 0.08$). CEB and residence show inverse correction with awareness related to STDs, the same is applicable to Beta value too. The table further indicates that CEB and husband's education determine significantly at 0.01 level and residence at 0.05 level, Beta value of each independent variable is presented in Figure 9.1.

The Beta value reflects the following predictions:

- Number of children ever born (CEB) shows negative determining impact on the awareness about STDs. More number of children ever born to a woman shows her

Figure 9.1
Regression Profile of STD Among Tribal Women

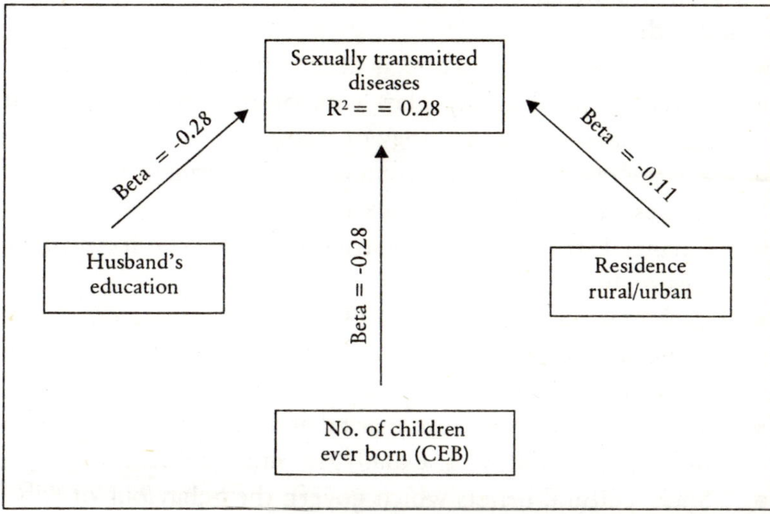

ignorance about appropriate family size, importance of sexual health and increases the beliefs related to high fertility and orthodox practices. All these variable restrict the woman from gaining knowledge about contagious and sexually transmitted diseases.

- Type of residence (rural/urban) contributes significantly to determine the awareness about STDs. Residential variations cause difference in availability and access to health care facilities. Rural inhabitants are comparatively more ignorant about sexually transmitted diseases.

Conclusion

The most obvious disadvantages faced by the tribal women are related to their health problems. Because of hilly areas and poor availability of medical facilities they suffer more in cases of sexually transmitted diseases. Socio-cultural and economic factors also influence several aspects of women's health in general and sexual health in particular. The sexual diseases are linked with faith in evil spirits and poor living conditions. It is concluded:

- Personal hygiene and effects of infection are overlooked.
- Illiteracy and poverty play a major role in shaping their ideas regarding the etiology of diseases.
- A large majority of the women avoid treatment because of shyness in revealing their sexual maladies.
- Financial stringency also restricts women to go for medical treatment.
- Lack of information about STDs and the consequent casual approach of the tribal women take a huge toll in terms of morbidity and mortality.
- The practice of *Nata,* pre-marital and extra-marital relations increase probability of sexually transmitted diseases.
- Socio-cultural beliefs which govern the behaviour of tribal women have great effect in the prevalence of RTIs, STIs STDs.
- Beliefs and practices of tribal women are associated with excessive faith in evil sprits, Jadu-Tona, Jhad-Phook, Jantra-Mantra and amulets, etc. They generally believe that evil spirits are responsible for all diseases.
- Nearly 80 per cent of all tribal women are aware about HIV/AIDS and its incurable nature. The awareness about RTI, STI and STD is three per cent, 14 per cent and 20 per cent respectively.
- Majority of tribal women believe that various diseases are a result of their sins of previous births.
- Lower the size of family, greater are the chances of utilisation of health facilities and prevention from STDs.
- Myths emerge as a important indicator in determining the various sexual complications. Lower the prevalence of myths in society, higher is the rational thinking, resulting in better health.

Suggestions

On the basis of findings, it is suggested that:

- Education is a key factor related to rational thinking. It is helpful in promoting health care. Educated male can play an important role in motivating women for adopting preventive and modern methods of treatment.
- Medical facilities available in urban areas should be expanded to tribal areas. This could be implemented through mobile dispensaries.
- For achieving low fertility and preventing STDs, greater use of contraceptives is needed. At policy level, decision should be taken to integrate medical treatment of STDs with Family Welfare Department.
- A large majority of the women avoid treatment because of shyness in revealing their sexual maladies to male doctors. Therefore, arrangement of lady doctors should be made for reproductive health and STDs check-up and treatment.
- Special health camps are required for diagnosis of the STDs and for imparting appropriate knowledge about STDs through audio-visual aids.
- For checking casual approach and myths of the tribal women towards STDs, the dangerous effects should be highlighted and advertised through traditional and modern means of mass communication.

References

Bhatia, Jagdish C. and John Cleland (1995) "Self-reported Symptoms of Gynecological Morbidity and their Treatment in South India", *Studies in Family Planning*, 26.

Bhende, Asha (1995) "A Study of Sexuality of Adolescent Girls and Boys in Underprivileged Groups in Bombay", *The Indian Journal of Social Work*.

Bryan (1994) *Human Sexuality*, Mayfield Publishing Company, Mountain View, California.

Centres for Disease Control and Prevention (1993) "Update: Barrier Protection Against HIV Infection and other Sexually Transmitted Diseases", *Morbidity and Mortality Weekly Report*, 42.

Chatterjee, Meera (1991) *Towards Better Health for Indian Women*, World Bank, South Asia Country Department II, Washington, D.C.

Chidambaram, R.N., Soorasangaran and S. Anbuganapathi (1986) "Morbidity Pattern in a Rural Community". *GIRH&FWT Bulletin*, 21.

Delaney, M. (1992) "Evidence Does Not Back Duesberg's AIDS Views", San Francisco, *Chronicle*, p. A14, September 4.

Goparaju, Laxmi (1993) "Unplanned, Unsafe: Male Student's Sexual Behaviour", paper presented at the workshop on sexual aspects of AIDS/STDs Prevention in India, Mumbai.

Nataraja, S. (1995) "Let's Get off the High Chair: AIDS and Women", *Voices*, No. 111, No. 2.

Osgood, C.E. et al. (1957), *The Measurement of Meaning,* University of Illinios Press.

Panthaki, D. (1998). *Education in Human Sexuality*: A source book for Educators, Mumbai. Family Planning Association of India.

Park, J.E. (1986), *Textbook of Preventive and Social Medicine*, Banarsidas Bhanot, Jabalpur.

Rao, N.S.N., S.M. Marwah, I.C. Tiwari, N.S. Murthy, V.M. Gupta and K.N. Dwive, (1973) "Disabilities, Morbidity and Mortality in a Community Development Block", *Indian Journal of Medical Sciences*, 27.

Turner, J.S. (1996) *Human Sexuality*, Prentice-Hall, Englewood Cliffs, New Jersey.

10

Sex Behaviour, Sexually Transmitted Diseases and Tribal Rajasthan

Mohammad Akram

The onslaughts of health hazards in the form of STDs/HIV/AIDS, which are sexually communicable complications, have added a newer dimension in the sexual life of the entire humanity, transgressing the boundaries of east and west or developed and underdeveloped. The sexually communicable infections (and diseases) have posed a great challenge to the entire generation to think differently about the "future of the present generation" and the "present of the future generation". Sex is no longer the personal affair of an individual; it has become the collective concern for the well-being of the entire humanity. Sex is no more an ethical or moral concern only; it has become a "physiological" and "clinical" concern, too.

The tribal society, besides being an integral part of the larger social structure, maintains some specific features in socio-

---

A short version of the article has been published in *Indian Journal of Sexually Transmitted Disease*, Vol. 26 No. 1, January-June, 2005.

cultural, spatial and historical terms. The tribal population, all over the world, is very vulnerable to the health hazards. Ethnographers, anthropologists and sociologists have given plenty of detail about sexual permissiveness among tribal populace. The customary practices and historical traditions continue to guide the normative structure related to sexual life. Polygamy, a residue of the primitive and medieval culture, continues to find acceptance among the tribes and the law does not prohibit it, at least in India.

The liberal attitude, increasing contact with other cultures and migratory movements to look for new job opportunities have exposed the tribal people sexually to outside world and consequently, they are increasingly becoming victims of STDs/HIV/AIDS. Although no comprehensive data is available for the Indian tribes, but, the scattered references found in the works of the sociologists, anthropologists, and medical practitioners, present a very gloomy picture.

Rajasthan is having a fairly good tribal population. As per the 2001 census, the tribal population in Rajasthan is 12.56 per cent of the total population. Out of these, more than 90 per cent of the total tribal population is consisted of two main tribal communities – the Bhil and the Meena. The tribal communities in Rajasthan are not evenly distributed. The districts having fairly good tribal population are Banswara (72.3%), Dungarpur (65.1%), Udaipur (47.9%), Dausa (26.8%), Sirohi (24.8), Sawai Madhopur (21.6%) and Chittorgarh (21.5%). On the basis of concentration of the tribal population, Rajasthan can be divided in two parts – northern and southern Rajasthan. Southern Rajasthan is having higher concentration of tribal population. The tribal-dominated areas in southern Rajasthan are notified as Tribal Sub-Plan (TSP) area.

This study is oriented towards an understanding of the sexual behaviour patterns, prevalence of non-marital sex and their larger implications in the spread of sexually transmitted diseases (STDs) among the tribal population of Rajasthan.

Methodology

This is an epidemiological study conducted in three Panchayat Samitis of three districts of the Tribal Sub-Plan (TSP) area of Rajasthan, namely, Pratapgarh in Chittorgarh district, Sagwara in Dungarpur district and Dhariavad in Udaipur district. Every Panchayat Samiti has been represented by the urban population along with three surrounding tribal-dominated villages. Two main tribes of the region are Bhils and Meenas. The design of the study and the sampling method is mainly based on the Latin Square Method. The specific advantage of the method is the fact that it allowed us to include several variables together in the study. This is mainly an exploratory study and also takes help from the descriptive designs.

The sampling unit selected for the study is an individual who has some exposure to sexual behaviour, irrespective of his/her marital status. A total of 180 samples have been selected for this study which include equal numbers of unmarried, married and widow/widower/divorcee selected from both the sexes. Further, in occupational terms, the samples include the wage labourers, the agriculturists and the other salaried class. At the micro level, a purposive sampling has been done to reach to individuals with identified and desired backgrounds. The method has been used mainly to reach to a heterogeneous population who had sufficient exposure to sexual relations.

The primary data has been collected by making use of an interview schedule and the cases related to STDs have been separately studied through case study method. The STDs are generally diagnosed medically but the tribal populations of Rajasthan are not very comfortable in going through such clinical examinations. A syndromic approach has been adopted for this study to identify the various symptoms related to the

STDs. The respondents were asked about the presence of the various complications (symptoms) among them and those who acknowledged about the problem were included for the detailed case study.

Sexual Act, Sexual Behaviour and STD

The sexual activity of an individual may involve a variety of experiences, a portion of which may culminate in the event which is known as orgasm or sexual climax. Kinsey et al. (1948: 157) described six chief sources of sexual climax. These are self-stimulation (masturbation), nocturnal dreaming to the point of climax (without intercourse), true heterosexual intercourse, homosexual intercourse, and contact with animals of other species. There are still other possible sources of orgasm, but they are rare and never constitute a significant fraction of the outlet for any large segment of the population.

Sexual activities may be solitary, involving only the single individual or they may be socio-sexual, involving two or more individuals. Masturbation and nocturnal dreams are the two chief types of solitary sexual activity. Heterosexual petting, heterosexual coitus, and homosexual relationship are the three main types of socio-sexual activity (ibid:227). Further, socio-sexual activities (sexual contacts) includes all range of hetero-sexual or homosexual behaviour including genital, oro-genital, oro-anal and genito-anal contact (Kothari, 1998: 64).

There are some individuals who derive 100 per cent of their outlet from a single kind of sexual activity. Most persons regularly depend upon two or more sources of outlet; and there are some who may include all six of them in some short period of time. This number varies considerably with different age groups and with different social levels.

Although human beings have a built-in biological sex drive, their membership in groups shapes or gives direction to this drive. Because different groups have different expectations and different values, beliefs and patterns of behaviour, sexual behaviour and even desires, vary from one group to another. This principle applies not only to different groups around the world but also to different groups within the same society. Consequently, sexual desires and behaviours differ by gender, race, ethnicity, age, religious orientation and social class. And hence, sociologists place a greater emphasis on the social aspects of human sexuality. Further, human sexuality, in its social framework, is so intermingled with the institution of marriage that marriage becomes, very often, the focal point of all sexual studies.

Marriage marks an important transition in an individual's life, and the timing of the event can have a dramatic impact on a young person's health. While in many societies a man's/women's first sexual experience is likely to be with his/her spouse, in others the beginning of sexual activity is not so closely linked to marriage. Differing expectations regarding relationship and sexual behaviour and a society's way of adapting to change in these expectations can have a profound impact on adolescents, youths, their families and society as a whole. Cultures around the world have varying attitudes towards sexual activity among unmarried people. Further, even married people do find sexual exposure outside their marital union.

Marriage, as an institution, is almost universal. All sexual activities between the spouses (husband and wife) are known as "marital sex". Sexual activities, beyond the marital union, are "non-marital sex" and it includes both pre-marital and extra-marital sex. Further, there is great extent of intermingling between pre-marital and extra-marital sex. An unmarried male/female may have sex with a married female/male. In such case, the sexual act of the unmarried person is pre-marital but the act of the married person is extra-marital. An unmarried person may have sex with another unmarried person (of opposite sex) and in this case both the partners are having pre-marital sex. Similarly, a married person may have hetero-sexual relation with another married person (not his/her spouse) and in such case both the partners are having extra-marital sex. Thus, "non-marital sex" includes multiple patterns of partnership.

The significance of non-marital sexual relations and especially sexual intercourse depends upon the success or failure with which the couple avoids an unwanted pregnancy. It is much affected even by the fear of such a pregnancy. Among the educated and socially exposed people, who use contraceptives or other methods of controlling unwanted pregnancies, the incidence of non-marital pregnancies is phenomenally low. Those pregnancies that do occur almost invariably represent instances where contraceptives were not employed. In segments of the population which rarely use contraceptives, the frequencies of non-marital (mostly pre-marital) pregnancies are quite high.

With the decline in average age at menarche and the trend towards increased age at marriage, the length of time in which adolescents may experience pre-marital sexual activities, have influenced the cultural values that make pre-marital sexual activities more appealing and acceptable to adolescents. Worldwide, young men and women are increasingly attending schools together (or meeting at other platforms, like places of work), and this increased interaction may also contribute to the incidence of sexual relationship prior to marriage.

Sexually transmitted diseases (STDs) are ubiquitous and all-pervading. They are found among all classes and in both the sexes. They are communicable diseases, which are transmitted by an infected man or woman to his/her partner during sexual intercourse (National AIDS Control Organisation, 2000). They are relatively easy to contract and are serious and painful. These diseases are actually a group of diseases whose reservoirs are human, transmitters are human and sufferers are human. The causative agent adapts itself to changing ecology and continues its existence with adjustable bio-mechanisms. These STDs are also known as venereal diseases. Osler called venereal diseases the most formidable enemy of the human race, an enemy entrenched behind the strongest human passion and deepest social prejudices, still holds good in our country (Thappa, 2002: 67).

The term 'STDs' denotes more than 25 infectious organisms, along with dozens of clinical syndromes that they cause. Some of such diseases are like gonorrhea, syphilis chancroid, lympho granuloma venerum (LGV), donovanosis chlamydis infections, genital herpes, genital warts, pelvic inflammatory disease, and Hepatitis B/A (Park and Park, 1985: 361). And, AIDS is a new addition in the list. They cause substantial morbidity and mortality that reduces productivity and earnings. These diseases can cause abdominal pain, ectopic pregnancies, still births, spontaneous abortions and even cervical cancers among women and total infertility among both women and men. Babies born to parents afflicted with STDs may suffer blinding eye infections and acute pneumonia (Kanbargi and Kanbargi, 1996:30). Since young men and women in their prime working ages are affected by these diseases, it also has serious economic consequences. These diseases are closely related to social circumstances and human behaviour. People consider these diseases as something unmentionable and consequently try to hide them. In no other branch of medicine, the quack, both inside and outside the profession finds such fertile and profitable field of exploitation of the gullible public as in this area.

Even though STDs have existed from the time immemorial and their clinical manifestations reasonably clear cut, the advent of HIV infection is forcing certain changes. HIV itself being a sexually transmitted pathogen and by its capacity to alter the immune mechanisms important in the pathogenesis and natural course of STDs, the clinical picture of both are significantly altered by each other. The risk behaviour to STDs and HIV is same. The major difference is that in the HIV infection the entry of the organism (virus) is identified only much later. The incidence of risk behaviour in a community can never be assessed accurately, but STDs are easier to pick up and all STDs are proof of unhealthy sex. Thus, STD is a pointer which can be easily picked up pointing to HIV-prone behaviour. Reduction in the number of STDs, if properly documented, is an indicator of improvement of sexual health in a community.

STDs have been a neglected area in public health in most of the developing countries despite the overwhelming fact of their impact on health, particularly of women and new born. Women, especially young women, are more vulnerable than men to infection with an STD and to its complication (such as infertility, cancer and inflammatory diseases). For example, in studies in developing countries, up to 20 per cent of the pregnant women have been found to have gonorrhea or chlamydia, up to 21 per cent to have syphilis. However, in India 8 per cent women have gonorrhea and 4 per cent women have syphilis (WPM, 1998).

Biologically, women are more susceptible to most STDs than men, partly because of the greater mucosal surface exposed to a greater quantity of pathogens during sexual exposure. In addition, the risk of STDs, including HIV infection is greater, whenever mucose is damaged. As a result of such factors, most STDs including HIV infection are transmitted more readily from men to women than from women to men.

The factors that contribute to the higher rate of STDs, as well as HIV, in women are also related to economic and gender inequalities. In many developing countries, the fact that men migrate to cities for work results in concentrations of men away from their families with a demand for sexual services. Where culture expects women to be passive and subservient to men, women have little or no control over decision-making relating to sexuality, nor do they have control over the sexual behaviour of their male partners, or over the use of condoms for the prevention of STDs.

It is estimated that about 333 million curable cases of STDs worldwide occur every year, most of which are occurring in developing countries (WHO, 1995). Globally, the AIDS epidemic has caused over 20 million deaths since it began and has orphaned more than 14 million children. With no available cure in sight, 42 million people were living with HIV/AIDS at the end of 2002 (HIV/AIDS, 2003:5). This disease has ravaged families and communities and, in the hardest hit countries, has reversed decades of progress in public health, economic and social development, education and food security. In 2002, approximately five million new HIV infections and 3.1 million AIDS death occurred worldwide. Women accounted for two million new infections and 1.2 million AIDS death in 2002. The number of people living with HIV/AIDS in India is approaching five million. The country has the second largest number of people living with HIV/AIDS, after South Africa. The percentage of adults (15-49) with HIV/AIDS in India is 0.8 (ibid: 6).

Review of Studies

Inhabitants of the Trobriand Islands encourage pre-marital sex, as it is thought to be an important preparation for marriage. In Asia the Lepcha society believes that girls need sexual intercourse in order to mature (Gagnon and Henderson, 1975: 10). Eskimos have a social custom which encourages husbands to offer male guests the privilege of spending the night with their wives, and it is considered a serious insult for guests to refuse. Further, some sub-cultures in Europe consider it appropriate for fathers to have intercourse with their daughters in order to teach them about sexuality (Zastrow, 1988:161).

Murthy (1993: xviii) opined that, in developing countries, pre-marital sex is sporadic and seldom recorded. However, the abortion records of the hospitals may give a clue to the prevalence of pre-marital sex in urban areas and villages surrounding urban hospitals. Further, in a country like India, pre-marital sex though prevalent in urban areas, it is difficult to record due to taboos on unmarried girls. Murthy further says that, in the present situation, some of the tribal population has such sanctions. He cites example of Murias of Bastar, who have youth dormitories which are very often used for pre-marital sex training. This system is also found in some other tribes, viz., Nagas of Assam, Santals of West Bengal and Bihar, the Oraons, Mundas and Birhors of Bihar (now Jharkhand), the Kharies, Juangs of Orissa, Mannans and Paluyans of Travancore.

Bhandari (1989: xv) observes that a Bhil woman is freer in sexual maters than Hindu caste woman. Mann (Bhandari 1989: xvi) also notes that the Bhils, under their customary law, do not consider sex indulgence, in case of unmarried boys and girls as a social offence. Nagda (1992) finds that the tribals of Rajasthan are generally more liberal to sex, than the other castes. Doshi (1971) found that a Bhil youth gets enough time for fun and frolic, while he is in jungle (forest) to graze his cattle and to watch the field. Malvi (1980: 37) mentions that according to records of General Hospital, Dungarpur, out of 100 outdoor patients, 2.2 are venereal disease cases. However, the figure given by Malvi is not tribal specific.

Akram (2005) states that the tribal communities of southern Rajasthan are exposed to the symptoms related to the STDs although they are not very aware of the terms like 'STDs'. A great number of them are not aware of the true causes of spread of the diseases. They are reluctant in taking specific precautions even after realisation of the problem. They are not much aware of the dire consequences of these diseases. Many among them have heard of AIDS which is the most deadly complication in modern context. But most among them are unable to link the STDs with AIDS.

Findings of the Study

This study, on the basis of the empirical findings, has tried to understand the very specific sexual practices and preferences prevailing among the tribal population of Rajasthan. Here, we will discuss some of the findings of the study.

Most Preferred Sexual Act

Table 10.1 presents the most preferred sexual act of the tribal people. Sexual intercourse is the most preferred sexual activity among the tribal people. However, the males express their sexual preferences more explicitly than the females as about one-fourth of the females have not mentioned about their preferences. Further, kiss and hugging are also preferred sexual acts among the tribal people, but by few only.

Table 10.1
Preferred Sexual Act

(in percentage)

Most preferred sexual act	*Males (N=90)*	*Females (N=90)*	*Total (N=180)*
Kiss	11.11	4.44	7.78
Sexual intercourse	72.22	60.00	66.11
Hugging	11.11	11.11	11.11
Not applicable/don't say	5.56	24.44	15.00
Total	100.00	100.00	100.00

Frequency of Sexual Intercourse between Marital Partners

Table 10.2 presents the frequency of sexual intercourse between the marital partners. It reflects that a little less than half of the respondents (42.22% males, 53.33% females) say that the normal frequency of sexual intercourse between married partners is two times in a week. One-fourth of the males say that it is not necessary to have sex (with wife) every week. About 92 per cent females want to have sex at least once every week but only 74 per cent males think like the females. Thus, the tribal women want to have more sex than their male counterparts, at least within the marital unions.

Table 10.2

Frequency of Sexual Intercourse between Marital Partners

(in percentage)

Frequency of sex	*Males (N=90)*	*Females (N=90)*	*Total (N=180)*
Once a week	14.44	18.89	16.67
Twice a week	42.22	53.33	47.78
Three or more times in a week	16.67	18.89	17.78
Not every week	25.55	2.22	13.89
Can't say	1.11	6.67	3.89
Total	100.00	100.00	100.00

Marriage and Sexual Relations

Table 10.3 presents the responses of the respondents regarding the belief that marriage is not necessary for establishing sexual relations. A little more than half of the respondents (56.67% males, 48.89% females) do not agree (fully disagree or disagree) with the statement that marriage is not necessary for sexual relations and 22.23 per cent (25.56% males, 18.89% females) say that they are agree (fully agree or agree) with it. Thus, for a little more than one-fifth of the population, sexual relation is not a privilege of only marital unions. Sex without marriage is of two types – pre-marital sex and extra-marital sex. This statement does not distinguish between pre-marital sex and extra-marital sex. It just talks about non-marital sex.

Table 10.3

Marriage is Not Necessary for Establishing Sexual Relations

(in percentage)

Opinions	*Males (N=90)*	*Females (N=90)*	*Total (N=180)*
Fully disagree	5.56	18.88	12.22
Disagree	51.10	30.00	40.55
Undecided	17.78	32.22	25.00
Agree	17.78	13.34	15.56
Fully agree	7.78	5.56	6.67
Total	100.00	100.00	100.00

Number of Known Males Having Non-marital Sex

Table 10.4 presents an estimation of prevalence of non-marital sex among the males. When the respondents were asked about their own experience of pre-marital and extra-marital sexual relations, most of them denied answering especially the females. When they were asked indirectly as how many of their known persons (males and females separately) are having such relations, the respondents replied without any hesitation. About 30 per cent (37% females, 22% males) of them said that they did not know any such males. The remaining 63 per cent of females and 78 per cent of males said that they knew at least

Table 10.4

Number of Known Males Having Non-marital Sex

(in percentage)

Known males	*Males (N=90)*	*Females (N=90)*	*Total (N=180)*
One	25.55	31.11	28.33
Two	26.67	23.33	25.00
Three or more	25.56	8.88	17.22
None/can't say	22.22	36.68	29.45
Total	100.00	100.00	100.00

one such male who is having such non-marital sexual relation. A quarter of the respondents say that they can identify two such males, and the next 25 per cent of the males can identify three or more such males who are having these relations.

Number of Known Females Having Non-marital Sex

Table 10.5 presents an estimation of prevalence of non-marital sex among the females. When asked about the females, one-fourth of the respondents said that they did not know any such females who are having non-marital sexual relations. The remaining 70 per cent males and females say that they can identify at least one such female who is having non-marital sexual relations. Amongst the females, 25 per cent say that they know three or more such females who get indulged in this sort of relationship.

Table 10.5
Number of Known Females Having Non-marital Sex

(in percentage)

Known females	*Males (N=90)*	*Females (N=90)*	*Total (N=180)*
One	32.22	16.66	24.44
Two	25.56	32.22	28.89
Three or more	17.78	25.56	21.67
None/can't say	24.44	25.56	25.00
Total	100.00	100.00	100.00

Thus, Tables 10.4 and 10.5 reveal that more than 70 per cent of the respondents can identify such males and females who are having pre-marital or extra-marital sexual relations. These tables, although do not give us the exact magnitude of those who have non-marital sex, but definitely suggest that such relations are very common and easily identifiable.

Community Opinion About Pre-marital Sex

Table 10.6 presents the opinion of the tribal people about pre-marital sex. Non-marital sex is generally a taboo in conservative societies and even in liberal societies, if it is not very permissive. The tribal people are not so conservative. When asked about opinion of the community about pre-marital sex about 40 per cent of the respondents say that it should not happen or it should be prohibited. About 14 per cent show their inability in expressing their views. The remaining 46 per cent of the respondents give some or other explanation for prevalence of pre-marital sex and the probable reasons for it. About one-fifth of the males and females think that it happens because of emotional ties between the would-be-spouses. A good number of tribal youths meet their would-be-spouse frequently and stay with them for quite some time. Very few females think that the pre-marital sexual relations are meant to know the health and sexual capacity of the would-be-spouses. A little more than one fifth of the females and one ninth of the males think that pre-marital sex is either meant for getting physical pleasure or it is by deceiving or out of greed. Thus,

Table 10.6

Community Opinion About Pre-marital Sexual Relations

(in percentage)

Community opinion about pre-marital sex	*Males (N=90)*	*Females (N=90)*	*Total (N=180)*
To know the would be spouse well	22.22	20.00	21.11
To know about the physical health and sexual capacity of the would be spouse	15.56	2.22	8.89
It should be prohibited	36.67	42.22	39.44
Can't say	14.44	13.33	13.89
For physical/carnal pleasure only	2.22	11.11	6.67
It is always by deceiving	8.89	11.11	10.00
Total	100.00	100.00	100.00

there is no homogeneous explanation for pre-marital sex-although the tribal societies appear to have a good degree of tolerance for pre-marital sex.

Remarriage/Nata

Table 10.7 presents the prevalence of second or third marriages in the form of *nata*. More than one-third of the respondents (more females than males) say that they can identify such persons in their community whose spouse got married to someone else during their absence for some or the other reasons. The respondents in almost every area that has been studied identified few such cases. Thus, the phenomenon of leaving one's spouse during his/her absence and start living with someone else (in the form of *nata*) is quite common among the tribal people although the magnitude of the event is not known. The practice of *nata* is an institutionalised form of extra-marital sexual relationship. However, among the tribal people, *nata* is not considered extra-marital sexual relationship as a female can have nata with some male only after ending her earlier marital tie although no formal process of breaking up the marital union (in the form of divorce) is required. However, for a male, break up of the marital tie is not necessary for bringing some other female through *nata*.

Table 10.7
Second/Third Marriage/Nata

(in percentage)

Second/third marriage/nata	*Males (N=90)*	*Females (N=90)*	*Total (N=180)*
Yes	27.78	43.33	35.56
No	50.00	51.11	50.56
Can't say	22.22	5.56	13.89
Total	100.00	100.00	100.00

Extra-marital Sex and its Impact

Table 10.8 presents the wide range of reactions of one spouse when the other is involved in extra-marital sex. Reactions to extra-marital sexual relations of the spouse are very different for two sexes. One-fourth of the females think that if their husband get involved in sexual relations with some other females then there is no way out for them but to get a divorce. Another one-fourth does not think of divorce but are sure that it will lead to quarrel and violence within the family. Thirty per cent of males and one-sixth of the females show a tit for tat treatment and say that as a reaction, even they will have such relations or bring/go for *nata*. A little less than one quarter of the respondents (29% of males, 17% of females) believe that they will maintain their marital ties and will try to bring change/correction in the behaviour of the spouse.

Table 10.8
Reaction to Extra-marital Sex of Spouse

(in percentage)

Reaction to extra-marital sex of spouse	*Males (N=90)*	*Females (N=90)*	*Total (N=180)*
Divorce	7.78	24.44	16.11
As a reaction, having sexual relation with someone else	15.56	15.56	15.56
Quarrel/violence with spouse	13.33	26.67	20.00
Trying to change the behaviour of spouse	28.89	16.67	22.78
No reaction/makes no difference	5.56	0.00	2.78
Having more sexual relations with the spouse	14.44	2.22	8.33
Any other/can't say	14.44	14.44	14.44
Total	100.00	100.00	100.00

Sex for Monetary Gains

Table 10.9 presents the responses of the respondents when they were asked whether they are acquainted with a female who can have sex for monetary gains. More than one-fourth of the respondents say that they know some person from their community who can have sex with others for monetary gains. Thus, according to the respondents, there are a good number of tribal women who can sell sex for monetary gains but such selling is done at individual level, in a personalised way and in clandestine manners.

Table 10.9

Acquaintance with Females who can have Sex for Monetary Gains

Response	*Number*	*Per cent*
Yes	49	27.22
No	104	57.78
Can't say	27	15.00
Total	180	100.00

Reasons of Commercial Sex

Table 10.10 reflects responses to a question related to reasons of commercial sex – by individuals, as well as, by the community. About one-fourth of the respondents said that it is a source of earning for those who, otherwise, have no other source of income. This segment of the population thinks that those who practice commercial sex are unable to work as wage labourers or as agriculturists. They cannot get any other source of earning livelihood and hence sell sex. Another 23 per cent think that this is very rewarding as it helps the commercial sex workers (CSWs) to earn good money as well as other rewards, in the form of gifts and favours. Another 18 per cent consider it as a profession. Thus, more than two-thirds of the respondents relate prostitution with economic gains and subsistence needs. About 10 per cent of the respondents think that it is a matter of personal choice of the concerned persons – and hence, prostitution is not an economic compulsion for them but a matter of preference.

Table 10.10

Reasons for Commercial Sex

Reasons	*Number*	*Per cent*
It is one of the professions	33	18.33
Because of no other source of earning	48	26.67
Traditional practice	29	16.11
Personal choice	17	9.44
Highly rewarding	41	22.78
Any other/can't say	12	6.67
Total	180	100.00

Reported Symptoms of STDs among the Tribal Population

Tables 10.11 and 10.12 state the variety of infections and symptoms reported by the female and male respondents respectively. The common symptoms for both the males and the females are related to sores, bumps, blisters on, in or near the genital organs followed by burning, itching and irritation in the genital organs. Some of the persons are suffering from single infection whereas many others are having multiple infections. From the medical point of view, STDs are curable if treated at earlier stages and otherwise they keep on multiplying the sufferings. Hence, a single patient carries multiple symptoms.

Table 10.11

Reported Symptoms of Females

Symptoms	*No. of respondents having each of the symptoms**
Bad smell from genital organs	3
Pain in the pelvic area between the naval and the sex organ	7
Burning, itching or irritation around the vagina	7
Bleeding from the vagina even without menstrual period	4
Pain deep inside the vagina during sexual intercourse	4
Sores, bumps, blisters on, in or near the genital organ	9
Burning and pain during urinating	7

*one person may report more than one symptom.

Table 10.12
Reported Symptoms of Males

Symptoms	*No. of respondents having each of the symptoms**
A drip or discharge from the penis	5
Sores, bumps, blisters on, in, or near the genital organ	12
Burning and pain during urinating	7
Painful ejaculation	2
Swelling of the penis	3

*one person may report more than one symptom.

Source of Transmission of STDs

Table 10.13 gives details about the probable sources of such infections among the patients studied. STDs are sexually transmitted infections and hence the source of such diseases are always some other human being. Identifying the source was the most difficult aspect of the study. The patients were interrogated in many ways and inferences were drawn on the basis of information revealed by the respondents. The main source of such transmissible infections is either multiple partner sexual relationship or sexual relations with commercial sex workers.

Table 10.13
*Main Source of Transmission as Identified by Respondents**

Source	*Males*	*Females*
Developed long back and you don't remember the source	4	6
Because of sex with unknown person	12	9
Sex with a person having the disease	6	5
Sex with commercial sex workers	7	0
Transmitted from spouse who was having the disease	3	4

*one person may identify more than one source.

Emergence of the Problem

Table 10.14 presents the timing of the first emergence of the problem. Most of the youngest are among those who have realised the problem in the current year. Contrary to it, among the aged persons most are those who have been realising the problems since last two-three or more years. All of the widow/widower/divorcee persons are among those who have these problems since last three or more years. Majority of the never married persons have realised the problem in current year. No significant difference is observable at gender level as the males and females are having a similar percentage distribution.

Table 10.14
First Emergence of the Problem

(in percentage)

First emergence of the problem	*Males (N=17)*	*Females (N=19)*	*Total (N=36)*
Present year	17.65	21.05	19.44
One year before	29.41	5.26	16.67
Two years before	17.65	26.32	22.22
Three or more years before	35.29	47.37	41.67
Total	100.00	100.00	100.00

Sharing the Problem with Spouse

Table 10.15 reflects sharing of the problem with the spouses. The never married persons do not have spouses and all of them are among those who have never informed spouses about the problem. None of the infected persons have told their spouse about the problem just after realisation of the problem. Thus, it can be certainly said that the infected persons felt it very difficult to share the problem with their spouses. Further, more than one-fourth of them did not tell about the problem, ever, to their spouses. The widow/widower/divorcee is among those who hide the problem the most (even then when they were having their spouse). In most of the cases, the spouse got to know about it himself/herself. Thus, there is a very visible divide between the husband and the wife about sharing the problem related to STDs.

Table 10.15
When Informed Spouse about the Problem

(in percentage)

Sharing problem with wife	*Males (N=17)*	*Females (N=19)*	*Total (N=36)*
Never	41.18	42.11	41.67
First year	0.00	0.00	0.00
Second year	5.88	10.53	8.33
Third year	17.65	26.32	22.22
Four and more year	35.29	21.05	27.78
Total	100.00	100.00	100.00

Table 10.15 also suggests that not sharing or informing about the problem to the spouse is one of the most important causes of spread of STDs as the spouse is the most vulnerable person in becoming victim of STDs once the other spouse has got it as they are, generally, the most regular sex partners. If, the husband or wife tell about the problem to his/her spouse immediately after realisation of the problem, then, the transmission to the spouse could be avoided.

Both Spouses Having Such Problem

Since STDs are sexually communicable, it is very likely that the infection will get communicated from the infected person to their spouses if the spouses are regular sex partners. The researcher also tried to interview the spouses of those who were identified to have some symptoms. About 40 per cent of such respondents, who reported to have symptoms of STDs, were unmarried and another one-fourth was either widow/widower or divorcee. Only one-third of such respondents were having regular sex partners in the form of spouses (wife or husband).

Among the seven married females who were identified to have such symptoms, two did not tell anything about their husbands, two said that they did not have any such problem or at least they did not know about it, and three said that they are also suffering from such problems. Out of these three husbands, one could not be contacted and the two others were included among the respondents.

Among the five married males who were identified to have the problem, four acknowledged that their wives are also having similar problems. Two out of these four females have already been interviewed and the other two females could not be interviewed because their husbands did not allow it.

Meaning of Safe Sex

Table 10.16 reflects the level of general awareness about safe sex among those who have reported to have the symptoms. The level of awareness is very low as more than 70 per cent males

Table 10.16

Meaning of Safe Sex

(in percentage)

Meaning of safe sex	*Males (N =17)*	*Females (N =19)*	*Females (N =36)*
No sex at all	0.00	5.26	2.78
Low frequency of sex	5.88	5.26	5.56
Sex with only known persons	35.29	21.06	27.77
Sex with only spouse	23.53	36.84	30.56
Using contraceptives during sex	29.42	26.32	27.77
Family planning	5.88	5.26	5.56
Total	100.00	100.00	100.00

and about 75 per cent females are not aware of the concept of "safe sex". About one-third of the males and one-fifth of the females consider sex with known persons as "safe sex". For 36.84 per cent females, sex with spouse is safe sex. Thus, most of them have no idea about the fact that use of condoms and contraceptives can protect them from transmission of the STDs.

Source of Treatment of STDs

Table 10.17 reflects the state of health facilities enjoyed by the tribal population. Only 31 per cent female patients and 41 per cent male patients are in touch with allopathic, ayurvedic or homeopathic doctors. Most of the patients either contact quacks and faith healers or get no treatment at all.

Table 10.17
Source of Treatment of STDs

(in percentage)

Source of treatment	*Males (N =17)*	*Females (N =19)*	*Total (N=36)*
Allopathic doctors	11.76	21.05	16.67
Homeopathic doctors	5.88	0.00	2.78
Ayurvedic doctors	23.53	10.53	16.67
Local practitioner/quacks	29.41	15.79	22.22
Faith healers (Bhopa/Dewra, etc.)	11.76	31.58	22.22
None	17.66	21.05	19.44
Total	100.00	100.00	100.00

Precautions Taken after Realisation of the Problem

Table 10.18 reflects use of contraceptives (condoms) is very low (5.8% among males and nil among females) among the infected persons. Further, only 29.4 per cent males and 26.3 per cent females continue with the medical treatment after diagnosis of the problem. About 20 per cent males and 42 per cent females maintain no precaution in their sexual behaviour mainly because of their perception that these infections are not serious and are very common.

Table 10.18

Precautions Taken After Realisation of the Problem

(in percentage)

Precautions taken	*Males (N =17)*	*Females (N =19)*	*Total (N=36)*
No precaution	29.41	42.11	36.11
Controlled/balanced sexual relations	17.66	10.53	13.89
No sexual relation with person other than spouse	5.88	10.53	8.33
Use of condoms during sexual relations	5.88	0.00	2.78
Medical treatment and medicines	29.41	26.30	27.78
Stopped all sexual relations	11.76	10.53	11.11
Total	100.00	100.00	100.00

Discussions

Sex and sexual relations are integral parts of tribal social structure. Sex is neither a taboo nor an inhibition for them and hence it enjoys a central position in the lives of the tribal population of Rajasthan. Sex is not only a state of mind but it exists as a physical reality in the day-to-day life of common tribal people. Sex is not always confined to the marital ties and it does exist before or beyond it. Sex before marriage in the form of pre-marital sex and sex beyond marriage as extra-marital sex are also realities in the tribal world. However, level and degree of acceptance for pre-marital and extra-marital sex varies in terms of the various sub-groups within them. Pre-marital sex is considered more acceptable than extra-marital sex.

Further, the tribal people are also exposed to commercial sex. Many males among them used to visit the commercial sex workers, whereas some of the tribal females also work as casual sex workers. The changing economic scenario and migration for new work opportunities have also exposed them to new sexual contacts. The changing scenario, have gradually exposed the tribal people to the sexually transmitted diseases.

The STDs, besides being biological, are also social in nature. The spread of these diseases depend upon the sexual contacts and hence, the network of social relations is also involved in their spread. The sociological enquiry of the problem largely involves the transmission pattern of the diseases and hence, the focus of the study is also the sexual contact tracing.

The empirical findings of the study reveal that the tribal population of southern Rajasthan is exposed to the symptoms related to the STDs although they are not very aware of the terms like STDs. A great number of them are not aware of the true causes of spread of the diseases. Further, the prevalence rate of STDs among all the respondents is 20 per cent. However, such prevalence includes only self-reported symptoms by the respondents and the statistics is not based on hospital reports. This reflects that a very high percentage of tribal people are having some or the other complications related to STDs. The source of transmission of such problems, as identified by the respondents, is mainly non-marital sexual relations. However, for some, the source is the spouse, who might have got the problem through non-marital sex with someone else.

The tribal population is exposed to both modern and traditional methods of treatment. But they prefer the traditional methods as their natural choice and go for modern methods only as the last choice. They are reluctant in taking specific precautions even after realisation of the problem. They are not much aware of the dire consequences of these diseases. A good proportion of them does not know the meaning of safe sex and hence are mostly unable to opt for the preventive methods.

Towards Sociology of Sexual Behaviour and Spread of STDs

The empirical findings, as delineated above, earnestly emphasise the need to look for a sociological framework to discuss the various intermingling aspects related to the sexual behaviour and spread of sexually transmitted diseases (STDs) among the tribal population. The sexual behaviour of the tribal population has been generally studied from the "evolutionary perspective". Some other studies have also seen the phenomenon from "cultural contact" perspective. The problems related to STDs are generally studied from the clinical and medical perspectives. Further the role of medicines and other treatment patterns have also been studied from the "diffusion" perspective.

The researches related to the present problem are at the crossroad. It still needs a specific direction. An all inclusive approach is yet to be developed. It is being realised by the present researcher that there is a need to develop an integrated approach to study the sexual behaviour and related problems and especially the problems related to the STDs.

The findings of the present study supplemented by the findings of other related studies which have been reviewed and incorporated at different stages by the present researcher, give the impression that the plethora of the problems related to tribal sexual life can be best expressed by the contrasts of "tradition" and "modernity" framework. At a different level, this can also be seen as the contrast between "ethnicity" and "modernisation". At a more generalised level, it can be said that the problems surrounding the tribal sexual life are mainly related to the problems related to "non-synchronisation" of "continuity" and "change" in tribal life. Thus, the present study pleads for the "continuity and change" model for studying the various aspects related to sexual life and spread of STDs among the tribal population.

More than five decades of planned change and more than two centuries of contact with modernity have influenced almost all the dimensions of life of the Indian population including the tribal population. Change, either in the form of "progress" and "development" or "transformation" has definitely created means as well as ends to move towards "modernity" or "globalisation" at a generalised level. The new means of communication and transportation are breaking the boundaries imposed by geographical or spatial limitations. On the other hand, the institutional structure including the norms, values, beliefs, customs and traditions has always been trying to maintain the "traditional" or the "ethnic" views of life. The transaction from "traditional" to "modern" or from "ethnicity" to "global" is never unilinear and the impacts, for the larger society, are also non-homogeneous. Amidst these transactions, the tribal population, in the opinion of the present researcher, is trapped between the opposite and contrasting lifestyles.

The beliefs and values related to sexual life of tribal population are mainly regulated by the normative structure which is very traditional in its orientation. The liberal attitude towards sex and the gender friendly environment of the tribal people is also a part of this traditional orientation. The prevalence of non-marital (including pre-marital and extra-marital) sex is also an indication of the traditional or being more specific, the ethnic orientation of life. But these tribal people are unable to maintain this traditional or ethnic orientation in the physical-environmental spheres of life because of the larger interventions and interceptions coming from the entire surrounding. Being specific, the tribal communities have lost their traditional control and dependence over forests and ecological surroundings, which have simply devastated their simplistic economies of fully dependence on natural surrounding. The loss of the simple "production-consumption" pattern of economy forced the tribal people to move out from their traditional dwelling in search of new employment opportunities. Growing contacts with alien cultures and other non-tribal people influenced all dimensions of tribal life including their sexual life. The findings of this study reveal at micro level that sexual exposure with non-tribal people gradually resulted in transmission of STDs among the tribal people.

Further, the changing work situation of the tribal people and their gradual exposure to other cultures also exposed the tribal males and especially the single living labourers to the commercial sex workers (CSWs). The "continuity" of the liberal attitudes towards sex and the "change" in the socio-economic atmosphere, paved the path of tribal males to visit the CSWs. And consequently, the tribal males, because of absence of adaptation of the "condom culture" became easy victims of sexually communicable tracts known as STDs. And further, the continuity of the indigenous treatment systems including faith healing and folk medicines became a barrier in getting proper treatment of the STDs.

Such paradoxes related to continuity and change can be easily identified in many aspects of sexual life and other related dimensions of life of tribal people. Tribal people are not very willing to opt for the varieties of sexual acts like smooching, necking, petting, or even oral or anal sex because of lesser emphasis in such acts in their traditional framework. But exposure to the pornographic magazines, movies and other erotic sex symbols in their new socio-economic settings, motivate them to bring variety in their sexual life by going for variety of sex partners. This ultimately results in continuation of their preference for non-marital sex, keeping them more vulnerable and susceptible for STDs.

Thus, we can sum up the entire discussion by making a generalisation that the continuation of the traditional cultural life (including the beliefs, values and practices related to sexual life) of the tribal people and the changing socio-economic and geographical patterns of modern life have created a great number of paradoxes and ironies in the life of tribal people. Their adaptation to the newer ways of life is non-synchronised, in the sense that their traditional or ethnic orientation is not getting synchronised with the modern means of life. The continuation of illiteracy, poor economic status, poor health culture and poor infrastructure support are becoming the structural barriers in achieving modern lifestyles. The onslaught of fast spreading STDs is definitely a product of this paradoxical change in tribal lifestyle.

References

Akram, M. (2005) "STDs and the Tribal Population", *Indian Journal of Sexually Transmitted Diseases*, Jaipur, Vol. 26, No.1, pp. 17-22. http://medind.nic.in/ibo/t05/i1/ibot05i1p17.pdf

Bhandari, B. (1989) *Tribal Marriages and Sex Relations*, Udaipur, Himanshu Publication.

Doshi, S.L. (1971) *Bhils: Between Societal Self Awareness and Cultural Synthesis*, Delhi, Sterling.

Gagnon, J. and Henderson (1975) *Human Sexuality: The Age of Ambiguity*, Boston, Little Brown.

HIV/AIDS in India (2003), Population Foundation of India, New Delhi.

Kanbargi, R. and Kanbargi, S., (1996) "STDs in Bangalore City: Some Findings From an Exploratory Study", *The Journal of Family Welfare,* 42;1, pp. 30-37.

Kinsey, A.C., et al. (1948) *Sexual Behaviour in the Human Male*, Philadelphia, WB Saunders Company.

Kothari, K. (1998) *AIDS,* Jaipur, A Rajasthan Medical Probe Publication.

Malvi, B.L. (1980) "Venereal Diseases in Dungarpur District", *Tribe* (Special Number), Vol. 12, No. 2-4, pp. 36-48.

Mehta, S., Groenen, R. and Roque, F. *Adolescents in Changing Times*, www.unescap.org/op/icpd/adoles.html, 1-22.

Murthy, M.S.R. (1993) *Sex Awareness among Rural Girls*, Delhi, BR Publishing Corp.

NACO (2000) Combating HIV/AIDS in India.

Nagda, B.L. (1992) *Social Correlates of Fertility*, Udaipur, Himanshu Publication.

Park and Park (1985) *Text of Preventive and Social Medicine*, Jabalpur, M/s Banarsidas Bhanot Publication.

Thappa, D.M. (2002) "History of Venereal Diseases and Venereology in India", *Indian Journal of Sexually Transmitted Diseases*, Jaipur, Vol. 23, No.2, pp. 67-79.

World Population Monitor (1998) *Selected Aspects of Reproductive Rights and Reproductive Health*, New York, UN.

Zastrow, Charles (1988) *Social Problems: Issues and Solutions*, Chicago, Nelson Hall.

11

Socio-Economic Profile of Sexually Transmitted Diseases Patients in Southern Rajasthan

Vani Verma

Sexually transmitted diseases (STDs) have severe consequences from the individual and community health point of view. Not only because of sequel but also because the risk of transmission of the human immuno-deficiency virus. They are a constant menace to the community health. Because of the social stigma attached to them, the cases are usually hidden and unreported in official records for the purpose of treatment. Sexually transmitted diseases, generally known as diseases spread by sexual intercourse, include syphilis, gonorrhea, genital warts, and genital herpes, etc.

Man is a social animal and does not live alone without having any relation with the world outside. Hence, social factors of the health are important as these factors play an active role in human body. There are some social factors, which makes an individual more vulnerable to indulge into risk taking behaviour and increase the risk of sexually transmitted diseases. These social factors include socio-economic status, occupation, educational status, type of family, religion, caste, marital status, knowledge, prostitution, sexual disharmony, etc. It can be seen that both medical and social factors play significant role in the context of sexually transmitted diseases.

In this study, efforts have been made to study the socio-economic profile of STD patients in urban and rural tribal societies. These factors include educational status, marital status, migration, socio-economic status, occupational status, attitude and knowledge regarding the diseases.

Methodology

The study was conducted in Udaipur division of Rajasthan state. This region is a part of tribal sub-plan area. It was carried out at department of skin and venereal diseases of Maharana Bhopal General Hospital, Aravali Hospital and Udaipur Hospital of Udaipur city. Efforts were also made to include Mahatma Gandhi Government Hospital, Banswara and Maharawal Government Hospital, Dungarpur. In these hospitals all the registered 180 STD patients and 80 HIV/AIDS patients were purposely selected for this study.

Keeping in mind the purpose and objectives of the study a comprehensive interview schedule for patients was designed. The patients of STDs/HIV/AIDS were taken into confidence and confidentiality of the information was assured. The collected data were classified, grouped, tabulated and analysed with the help of suitable statistical tool.

Findings and Discussion

Age

The age expressed by the patient on the day of interview was considered as the actual age of the patient and it was recorded in round figures. This way, the age of STD patients and HIV+ patients were recorded separately and the data are presented in Table 11.1 which shows that patients were categorised into three age groups, i.e., less than 25 years, 25 to 35 years and 35 to 45 years. The maximum number of STD patients was in the age group of 25 to 35 years (57.22%) followed by the age group of less than 25 years (28.89%). The least number of patients (13.89%) were of the higher age group, i.e., 35-45 years. The youngest STD patient recorded was 15 years and the oldest was 45 years of age (both were male).

Table 11.1

Distribution of Patients on the Basis of Age and Sex

Age (in years)	*STD Patients*			*HIV+Patients*		
	Male	*Female*	*(N=180)*	*Male*	*Female*	*(N=80)*
25-35	85 (47.22)	118 (10.0)	103 (57.22)	39 (48.75)	20 (25.00)	59 (73.75)
>-25	42 (23.33)	10 (5.56)	52 (28.89)	11 (13.75)	0 (0.00)	11 (13.75)
35-45	16 (8.89)	9 (5.00)	25 (13.89)	10 (12.0)	0 (0.00)	10 (12.50)
Total	143 (79.44)	37 (20.56)	180 (100.00)	60 (75.00)	20 (25.00)	80 (100.00)

Figures in parenthesis are percentages.

Similarly, the maximum number (73.75%) of AIDS patients recorded were of the age group of 25-35 years followed by patients of less than 35 years of age. Only 12.50 per cent were of 35-45 years of age. The youngest patient was of 20 years of age whereas the oldest one was of 45 years of age.

In this study it was recorded that the middle-age group patients, i.e., (21 to 25 years) were more vulnerable as compared to low and higher age groups patients.

Sex

The sex of STD and HIV+ patients was recorded to know the mode of infectious diseases and their ratio in the society. The data of Table 11.1 explains that 79.44 per cent males were infected by the STD and only 20.6 per cent females were infected by such diseases. But, in case of HIV+ patients, the number of males was 75 per cent whereas that of females only 25 per cent, which is relatively 4.4 per cent higher than that of STD patients. Kinsey (1953) reveals that venereal diseases are ubiquitous and all pervading. They are found among all diseases and in both the sexes.

This study also reveals that the male respondents were more vulnerable as compared to female respondents. The reason may be that men have more freedom than women. Men can take their own decision. In case of females, as it can be seen in every stage of life, they are dominated by the family members especially by the male members. Further, it was also observed that males engaged more in extra-marital relations as compared to females.

Majority of patients in our series hailed from urban areas as compared to rural areas because of urbanisation, modernisation, industrialisation, etc. They are two to three times more in cities. Most of the patients were in lower and middle income groups while only a few were from the higher class. It is common knowledge that STD is always higher in low socio-economic groups because of poverty, crowded living conditions, migration, lack of recreational facilities and cultural deprivation.

The literacy rate among the STD patients were recorded on a 7-point scale. Due to less frequency in some of the categories, the categories were finally pooled into 4 in number. It was found that the highest percentage of STD patients (Table 11.2) were illiterate (38.33%) followed by literate (21.66%) and the school educated were (26.11%). The least number of the patients were college students (13.88%).

Table 11.2
Distribution of Patients on the Basis of Education

Statement	*STD Patients*			*HIV+Patients*		
	Male	*Female*	*Total (N=180)*	*Male*	*Female*	*Total (N=80)*
Education						
Illiterate	49	20	69	20	10	30
	(27.22)	(11.1)	(38.33)	(25.00)	(12.50)	(37.50)
Literate	22	10	39	0	10	10
	(16.11)	(5.56)	(21.66)	(0.00)	(12.50)	(12.50)
School	40	7	47	35	0	35
	(22.2)	(3.89)	(26.11)	(43.75)	(0.00)	(43.75)
College	25	0	25	5	0	5
	(13.88)	(0.00)	(13.88)	(6.25)	(0.00)	(6.25)
Total	143	37	180	60	20	80
	(79.44)	(20.56)	(100.00)	(75.00)	(25.00)	(100.00)

Figures in parentheses are percentages.

Similarly, in case of HIV+ patients, it was found that 43.75 per cent were school educated, 37.50 per cent were illiterate, 12.5 were literate and only 6.25 per cent were college educated.

It can be concluded that illiterate people are more sensitive to sexually transmitted diseases as compared to the literate people. They are more vulnerable as compared to other groups, but it is also seen that even educated people were suffering from these diseases, even though they were well aware of such contagious diseases, but they did not use any protection against these diseases. Therefore, due to unawareness and carelessness, these diseases are rapidly spreading at a faster rate among people.

Occupation

The data of Table 11.3 represent that 38.89 per cent migrant labourers were STD patients followed by 16.67 per cent truck drivers/jeep drivers/auto drivers and khalasis. The data also report that 17.22 per cent STD patients were skilled labourers, 8.89 per cent businessmen, 18.33 per cent housewives and unemployed boys.

Table 11.3

Distribution of Patients on the Basis of Occupation

Occupation	*STD Patients*			*HIV+Patients*		
	Male	*Female*	*Total (N=180)*	*Male*	*Female*	*Total (N=80)*
Migrant labour	60 (33.33)	10 (5.56)	70 (38.89)	20 (25.00)	0 (0.00)	20 (25.00)
Unemployed	11 (6.11)	22 (12.22)	33 (18.33)	0 (0.00)	20 (25.00)	20 (25.00)
Drivers	30 (16.67)	0 (0.00)	30 (16.67)	32 (40.00)	0 (0.00)	32 (40.00)
Skilled labour	26 (14.44)	5 (2.78)	31 (17.22)	0 (0.00)	0 (0.00)	0 (0.00)
Business	16 (8.89)	0 (0.00)	16 (8.89)	8 (10.00)	0 (0.00)	8 (10.00)
Total	143 (79.44)	37 (20.56)	180 (100.00)	60 (75.00)	20 (25.00)	80 (100.00)

Figures in parentheses are percentages.

Similarly, in case of HIV+ patients it was found that 40 per cent were truck drivers/auto drivers/jeep drivers and khalasis. The per cent of migrant labours and business were 25 and 10 per cent. Vyas (1980) pointed out that the prevalence of STDs were more among high-risk group like migrant laboures, seamen, soldiers, unskilled labours and tourists.

It concludes that migrant labourers and drivers were more vulnerable as compared to other occupational groups like skilled labourers and businessmen. As these people move frequently outside and after living for some months or years return home with some STD/HIV/AIDS and they give this diseases to their wives and future generations.

Residential Location

Table 4 shows that the maximum numbers of STD patients were from urban areas (65%) as compared to the rural areas (35%). Similarly, in case of HIV+ patients, it was recorded that 72.5 per cent were from urban areas and 27.5 per cent were from the rural areas. It concludes that the STD and AIDS patients were more in the urban areas as compared to the rural areas.

Table 11.4

Distribution of Patients on the Basis of Residential Location

Residence	*STD Patients*			*HIV+ Patients*		
	Male	*Female*	*Total (N=180)*	*Male*	*Female*	*Total (N=80)*
Urban	87 (48.33)	30 (16.67)	117 (65.00)	43 (53.75)	15 (18.75)	58 (72.50)
Rural	56 (31.11)	7 (3.89)	63 (35.00)	17 (21.25)	5 (6.25)	22 (27.50)
Total	143 (79.44)	37 (20.56)	180 (100.00)	60 (75.00)	20 (25.00)	80 (100.00)

Figures in parentheses are percentages.

Family Type

Efforts were made in the study to identify the family structure of STD and HIV+ patients and the observed data are presented in table. The maximum number of STD patients were belonging to nuclear families (53.33%) followed by joint families (46.67%). Similarly, the maximum number of HIV+ patients were from nuclear families (65%) and only 36.25 per cent were from the joint families. It shows that nuclear family-structure provide situation to family members for indulging in promiscuous practices. Shendra and Tiwari (2002) reveal that the people living in nuclear families were at risk as compared to those living in joint families.

Table 11.5

Distribution of Patients on the Basis of Family Type

Type of Family	*STD Patients*			*HIV+ Patients*		
	Male	*Female*	*Total (N=180)*	*Male*	*Female*	*Total (N=80)*
Nuclear	79 (43.89)	17 (9.44)	96 (53.33)	40 (50.00)	12 (15.00)	52 (65.00)
Joint	64 (35.56)	20 (11.11)	84 (46.67)	21 (26.25)	8 (10.00)	29 (36.25)
Total	143 (79.44)	37 (20.56)	180 (100.00)	60 (75.00)	20 (25.00)	80 (100.00)

Figures in parentheses are percentages.

Marital Status

The data collected related to marital status of STD patients represent that the maximum number of respondent (69.44%) were married, followed by 24.4 per cent who were unmarried boys were infected by STD. The boys were street boys, college students, labourers and businessmen. It was pointed out that those 1.67 per cent girls were also STD patients who got infection from their friends. This table further indicates that 5.56 per cent widower found infected from this diseases. In case of HIV patients 50 per cent married male and 25 per cent female were found infected. It is also observed that 6.25 per cent unmarried boys were also infected from these diseases who were migrated labourers working at metropolitan cities. This table also indicates that 6.25 per cent widowers were infected with these diseases.

Table 11.6
Distribution of Patients on the Basis of Marital Status

Marital Status	*STD Patients*			*HIV+ Patients*		
	Male	*Female*	*Total (N=180)*	*Male*	*Female*	*Total (N=80)*
Married	92 (51.11)	33 (18.33)	125 (69.44)	40 (50.00)	20 (25.0)	70 (87.50)
Unmarried	41 (22.78)	3 (1.67)	44 (24.44)	5 (6.25)	0 (0.00)	5 (6.25)
Widow/widower	10 (5.56)	1 (0.56)	11 (6.11)	5 (6.25)	0 (0.00)	5 (6.25)
Total	143 (79.44)	37 (20.56)	180 (100.00)	60 (75.00)	20 (25.00)	80 (100.00)

Figures in parentheses are percentages.

In the study it was seen that more married people had STD as compared to unmarried and widows/widowers. It was observed that a number of female patients were brought to the clinic by their husbands who had given the disease to their spouse. It may be seen that promiscuous married males get infected by extra-marital relations and then pass it on to their wives.

Economic Status

The socio-economic status of the patients was recorded on the scale developed by Udai Pareek and G. Trivedi. On the basis of total obtained score by each patient, they were grouped with three categories with the help of SD low, medium and high socio-economic status.

The maximum number of STD patients were from lower category class, (i.e. 57.22%) followed by 38.89 per cent middle category and the least number of patient were of higher category. In case of HIV+ patients, it was found that the maximum number of patients were belonging to lower category (50%) followed by middle category (40%) and the minimum number of patients were of the higher category (10%).

Table 11.7
Distribution of Patients on the Basis of Socio-economic Status

Socio-economic Status	*STD Patients*			*HIV+Patients*		
	Male	*Female*	*Total (N=180)*	*Male*	*Female*	*Total (N=80)*
Low	71 (39.44)	32 (17.77)	103 (57.22)	10 (12.50)	30 (37.50)	40 (50.00)
Middle	56 (31.11)	5 (2.78)	61 (33.89)	32 (40.00)	0 (0.00)	32 (40.00)
High	16 (8.89)	0 (0.00)	16 (8.89)	8 (10.00)	0 (0.00)	8 (10.00)
Total	143 (79.44)	37 (20.56)	180 (100.00)	50 (62.50)	30 (37.50)	80 (100.00)

Figures in parentheses are percentages.

The finding concludes that majority of patients were from urban areas compared to rural areas because of urbanisation, industrialisation, modernisation of urban areas as they migrated from rural areas for employment. STD patients were more in low socio-economic group due to poverty, crowded living conditions, migration, lack of recreational facilities and cultural deprivation.

Conclusion

The present study shows that the majority of the patients were belonging to 25-35 year group. The chances of exposure of this group are also likely to be high and hence freedom and prevalence are usually found in such an age group rather than in other groups. The study has pointed out that males were more infected as compared to females, as males enjoy more freedom in all respects in the society as compared to females. The incidence of sexually transmitted diseases was higher in the illiterate as compared to the other groups. There were more cases of sexually transmitted diseases among low-income groups as compared to the other groups, and in sero-positive it was found that middle-income group people were more vulnerable as compared to other groups as the low-income group people had less migration to metropolitan cities as compared to middle class. The findings also show that the men living in nuclear families were more vulnerable as compared to joint families, as family restrictions are less and people face loneliness or frustration and due to sexual urge are more vulnerable to sexually transmitted diseases. The most prevalent group was the married, as compared to the unmarried and widows/widowers. The diseases were more prevalent in rural areas as compared to urban areas and mostly among the people who had migrated. As people usually migrated to urban sectors, on their return they bring such diseases with them and pass it on to their spouse and future generations. It seems that the urban diseases are being spread to the rural areas.

References

Kinsey, A.C. et al. (1953) *Sexual Behaviour in Human Female*, Philadelphia, WB Saunders Company.

National AIDS Control Programme, Phase-2 (Rajasthan).

NACO (2000-2—1), Combating HIV/AIDS in India, Govt. of India.

Shendra and Tiwari (2002) “Teens, Sex and AIDS” *AIDSASIA*, p.12.

Shukla, G.C. (2001) “HIV Background Report”, Udaipur Region, p.1.

UNICEF State Office, Rajasthan. Rajasthan State AIDS Control Society (2001). “HIV/AIDS in Rajasthan”.

WHO (2002), Website.

12

Sociology of Medicine for the Tribals

Balveer Singh

Medical sociology employs the perspectives of the general sociological constructs in the analysis of behaviour of groups in health and medical services. Such an approach to society is relevant when we discuss the medical and health situation of our Indian society. It is well known that no society can achieve economic development until such time that the health of its people is properly and adequately taken care of. The providers of community health services have to carefully identify the health needs of the people and to man the services in such a manner as to provide integrated health care to the individual, the family and the community.

The health needs of the people are related to the community social structure and it changes according to the changes observed within the structure. The health behaviour of a Bhil therefore, is determined by the attitude, motive and normative pattern often influenced by the social, cultural and economic factors operating within and without the social structure of the community or society. The ethno-methodology of the people therefore, goes a long way in providing shape to the working of health and medical services. It is the ethno-methodology which provides motivational aspects related to the preventive or curative medical and health care. And therefore, it also becomes obligatory for the health care system to come to the expectations of the people and these are also influenced mostly by the social, cultural, economic and situational factors in the community. The Bhils are nourished in a situation of protective discrimination. The development plans have created increasing awareness and consciousness among them. The Bhils therefore, look at the government as the provider of health and medical care for certain specialised services, or to the availability of minimal and medical care at their doorsteps. The incidence of different diseases, factors of causation, notification and preventive and curative measures constitute an important aspect of the management and organisation of health services in a country, but the interaction of these sets of factors with the physical and the cultural environments is crucial in designing health and medical care services to the changing social structure of the country or the community.

Theoretically speaking, the concept of health or illness becomes institutionalised within the social and cultural milieu of each community and its level of development, in other words, one measure of social development could be cultural conception of illness. The tribals relied more on their instincts to stay healthy and since they could not largely comprehend the functioning of the human body, magic became an integral part of their beliefs about the causes and cures of health disorder. Despite the progress made in public health through improved hygiene and sanitary living conditions, and development of germ theory of diseases through bacteriological researches for combating diseases and restoring normalcy, their belief in some magic or religious power involving forces beyond human comprehension is still being held not only in India but in most of the developing countries.

Most of the studies conducted in the realm of medical sociology are primarily exploratory and to some extent diagnostic in nature. Many of these are sketchy in nature and provide gaps to be filled in regard to the knowledge, belief and practice status of people related to causation, curation and prevention of diseases. Notwithstanding the methodological attempt to study these problems, they have thrown up a number of hypotheses which need to be validated in different geographical and cultural regions of the country for developing a coherent theory on "health and disease".

Our objective of studying the medical sociology in its various aspects among the Bhils is based on the very often advanced observation prevalent among planners, administrators, and members of middle class that the Bhils, quite like the other socially disadvantaged groups, survive on erroneous concepts about health and diseases. It is alleged that they are highly superstitious. They are buried in ignorance, illiteracy and backwardness. They would never accept innovations in medical cure. This widely held and occasionally strengthened observation was found to be erroneous by us in the field.

The Bhils who constitute about 12 per cent of the general population of the State are found mostly in the southern districts administratively covered by the tribal sub-plan area of the state. Though the Bhils have migrated from their homeland-hills and forests, during last hundred years, they have migrated to plains also. Those of them who have migrated and have been living in the city from two to three generations, are found caught between their traditional method of treatment and the allopathic method.

The traditional medical structure possesses all the aspects of a medical system. They have traditional methods of diseases prevention. There are some foods which are considered to be "cold" and some to be "hot". Lemon is taken to be "cold" beverage which causes cold and cough. Similarly, eggs are considered to be hot and are therefore, avoided during summer.

The Bhils provide treatment in illness through medical herbs, plants and leaves. The elder men of the village are familiar with some of these herbal medicines. In illness these medicines are applied. However, if the traditional herbal treatment fails, they take recourse to magic and charms. There are Bhopas (the magic man) who practice the therapy of magic. If this system of cure also fails, there is option to approach the allopathic system. What we want to make is that despite the tribal living in the urban neighbourhoods, they are quite familiar with the indigenous methods of treatment. It appears that even in future, with the Bhils getting more and more modernised, the practice of their indigenous practice would not die. It is because that the Bhils have an abiding faith in their traditions which have strong historical depth.

The above discussion leads us to its corollary, namely, that if the Bhils continue to have some faith in traditional medicine, in the context of allopathic medicine, what aspects of allopathic medicine are getting weak. Empirical evidences show that the herbal medicines which used to be available to the Bhils in the hills and forests is now not available. First, with the decay of the forests, the medicinal plants and herbs have become non-existent. Second, the Bhils in the urban neighbourhoods are required to go to their original home to collect the medicinal plants. It becomes, therefore, a costlier affair. Similarly, there is dearth of persons in the urban neighbourhoods who are skilled to practice magic-charms and Bhopai – the art of possession and the rituals of hocus-pocus. Despite having some faith in the traditional system of medicine, the Bhil in the neighbourhoods is required to abandon the practice of traditional medicine.

The Bhils and for that matter the tribals in general have a specificity of culture. Even though they are away from their traditional milieu of hills and forests, it is found that while living in the city they still suffer from their age-old nostalgia of depending on the treatment which is related to forests and food habits. This can be explained by the fact that the Bhils have sought their integration in the urban society only partially. They still share with others, those living in the rural plains and hills and forests, their primordial culture. As a matter of fact, the tribals have their socio-economic structure, they have their food choices, values from nutrition and they cherish a health status which very well corresponds to their style of living. When there is diffusion of innovation from the non-tribal society, besides the structural constraints, there are constraints of language and interaction. The Bhils in urban neighbourhoods, especially their women, have successfully learnt the working knowledge of Hindi which helps them to understand their job and places of work. But, the knowledge about technology, particularly medicine, which comes to them is not fully comprehended. These are some of the structural obstacles which come in their way.

What is interesting about the tribals of the urban neighbourhoods is that they do not have any structural institutions which could keep alive their faith in the traditional system of medical treatment. Lack of this, it may be argued, would lead to the total extinction of the traditional method of cure.

A new group of tribal fundamentalists has emerged which is concerned about the problem of the social and cultural identity of the tribals. These fundamentalists are actually revivalists. They argue that if the tribals do not maintain their primordial identity, there is possibility of the non-tribal civilisation to "eat up" their antiquity. And, therefore, in their line of argument they say that even if the tribals' old practices posses merit or not, they must be followed. That will provide a genuine base for their future social survival. This group, therefore, very strongly holds that the tribals may use allopathic medicine but at the same time they must stand for the perpetuation of their tradition which contains a glory for them. Their argument is further strengthened when they say that in the future when the government at some point of time withdraws the constitutional safeties and securities, the tribals would be left high and dry without any structure which they could claim to be their own. It is for this reason also that the traditional system of medicine has to be kept alive.

The empirical experiences suggest that the problem of the acceptance of allopathic medicine vis-à-vis traditional medicine is not taken by the tribals in the form of either this or that. It is not that the tribals who have accepted allopathic medicine have abandoned their traditional medicine. Nor is it correct to say that those who practice traditional medicine do not have any consideration for allopathic medicine. The situation therefore is very subtle. The tribals look to a variety of factors. They make access to a particular system looking to a large number of factors: economic, cultural and political. However, on the strength of data at our disposal, it could be stated without any reservation that the illness which requires surgical operations, is firmly considered to be an area where allopathic approach is the most suitable.

In the area of non-surgical treatment that is in the field of medicine the informants believe that they have some medicinal plants which are highly useful. The difficulty is that a large number of plants have now become extinct. Though, in the field of disease and cure, the tribals are today between their traditional medicine and the allopathic medicine, by and large, their society is favourably inclined towards the acceptance of allopathic medicine, provided they have money to spend on it. The tribals who are employed in government service consider allopathic medicine to be their first preferences – expenses on this account are met by the State government.

Much requires to be done in the field of personal hygiene and public health. A very cursory observation of the food habits, keeping up of the cleanliness of house, manners of taking food would show that the tribals lack considerably in the field of hygiene. Most of the inadequacies in their personal hygiene are due to poverty and lack of education.

In the area of public health, the situation is still worse. There is almost total absence of public urinals and latrines. People ease at any space which is not habitated by people. Further, water facility is also not adequate. The relative lack in personal hygiene and public health weakens the preventive aspects of tribal illness. It is in this area that municipal corporation and public health department can contribute substantially.

In the closing, it may be said that any system of medicine and also the incidence of illness are specific to a particular social structure. The tribal social structure, like other social structures, has its own structural and ethnic specificity. The diseases which inflict upon the tribals are likewise specific to the attributes of tribal social structure. Each disease, despite being pathology of human body, is also sociology of human society. Quite like the social aspects of illness, there are also social and cultural aspects of medicine. And it is on this hypothesis that we argue that the sub-discipline of medical sociology should construct and develop perspectives which should have bearing for the particular study of tribal society. Can this be done, constitutes an area of further research.

13

Our Ancient Wisdom

The Panacea of All Maladies (with Special Reference to STDS)

N.K. Jha

The topic of the present discussion appears to be most timely and appropriate because we are living in an age, where the impact of materialism is undoubtedly immense and has completely destroyed the ethical values, the sustainer of our way of life, our greatest heritage. We are living in a world which is dominated by greed and competition, speed and restlessness, pollution and ecological destruction. Man seems to have conquered both time and space. It has become feasible to explore other planets. Due to unprecedented scientific advancement, such new vistas have been opened that is simply miraculous. The world is bubbling with great success in every sphere and the speed studded with thrill is unparalleled. Man has achieved everything which he needs for the satiation of his unlimited yearnings, seemingly unaware of the harm and ill-effects generated in this suicidal process. But it is a very natural process because worldly beings long for happiness which they perceive to attain through fulfilment of never-ending desires. But desires, even if fulfilled, generate more desires.[1] Their intrinsic nature is to multiply like the branches of a tree which result in miseries of all sorts whether physical or mental all around. The laws of nature remain as it is but the perceptional lack of understanding in negotiating with them is the root cause for sufferings and miseries. This illusive perception, misconception and unawakenness give rise to false beliefs and false conducts. In this blind search for advancement and happiness mental and physical unrest has creeped into life. In this mad race of quenching the never-ending thirst, human being has forgotten ways to harmonise the outer and inner as well as to establish the desired equilibrium. No doubt, scientific development has enriched us and provided us with all outward comforts and pleasures but the very existence of mankind seems at the verge of extinction. In a nutshell, the present world seems to have reached the no-return point.

But we, as Indians, should not suffer within through a sense of remorse and repentance since we are gifted with invaluable legacy of knowledge (*Bhartiya Vidya*) studded in our ancient scriptures which offer remedial solutions for every ailment. So called "modern man" may naturally ask as to why in this Internet age we go back to old and outdated ideas of our scriptures. The justification for this retrospection is beautifully presented by Paul Brunton in his classic *The Spiritual Crisis of Man:* "Without inward peace, without outward security, modern man who for so long pitied his ancient and medieval fathers is now himself to be pitied." This is the picture of an average human being today. The scientific discoveries cannot negate the important purports of our age-old scriptures which have endured the test of time. Mahatma Gandhi had once said that the past belongs to us but we do not belong to the past. We cannot allow ourselves to be prisoners of the past. Nor can we afford to forget or neglect our precious past. We must, therefore, preserve and perpetuate the best of the past in the present and use its building blocks in raising the edifice of the future. So, we do not have any reason to stay bewildered with such a great heritage of scriptural gifts which are simply beyond the realm of scientific advancements. It is totally judicious and justified to retrospect for invaluable suggestions of our seer-ancestors, to look back to our scriptures for propitious instructions embedded in them besides modern scientific efforts to mitigate health hazards. Our scriptures, rooted in Vedic sources, carry the messages of the great spiritual masters, *rishis*, whose light of true wisdom can dispel ignorance and help stop the erosion of moral, spiritual and scientific values prevalent in the world today. It would not be any exaggeration to say that our yogis and rishis were true scientists who set examples of inquisitiveness and original research which is beyond the vision of modern scientists. It is not without reason that tension-stricken, strife-ridden and sunken in deep ocean of incurable maladies, West is turning to India for spiritual guidance and repose as well as meditational clues and Ayurvedic cures.

Human body is regarded as the most important means to attain highest physical and spiritual goals in life throughout our classical literature. *Caraka Samhita Nidana* says, "one must look after one's physical body first leaving other worldly things aside because in the absence of body, nothing will have existence."[2] The great poet Kalidasa also gives this clarion call in his celebrated epic *Kumara Sambham* when God Shiva as a celibate approaches Parvati who is indulged in 'Tapas'.[3] Another Ayurvedic text *Arogya Muktavali* suggests that one should be vigilant enough in protecting his body as the lord of the town remains vigilant in protecting his town, as the charioteer in protecting his chariot.[4] There are numerous suggestions scattered in our scriptures regarding the importance of stout physique.

Health has been defined as a state of dwelling in one's own pleasure-self *Svasmin Tisthatiti Svastha*...Furthermore, a complete definition of a healthy state of body or health has been furnished by Ayurvedic seer Susruta. According to him, a person having balanced temperaments (*Vatta, Pitta* and *Kapha*), having thirteen fires within as well as seven (*Dhatus*) constituent elements, uninterrupted outflow of residuals and whose soul, mind and organs are happy is called "healthy".[5] In other words, a person should be healthy physically, mentally as well as spiritually. The *Caraka Sutra* says that a physical body free from diseases, can attain the state of *Purusartha* – the ultimate pursuits, namely, *Dharma* – discharge of duty, *Artha* – acquirement of wealth, *Kama* – gratification and *Moksa* – the final emancipation.[6] WHO defines health as follows: "Health is a complete physical, mental and social well-being and not merely an absence of diseases or infirmity". This definition endorses the views expressed in above lines.

Vedic texts, particularly *Atharvaveda* and *Rgveda*, also mention various ailments and describe their treatments. Medicine was practised by priests as well as others conversant with it. Diseases were considered as a punishment against various human sins, inflicted by Gods directly or through various demons. The appropriate treatment was placating the irate Gods, fighting or driving out the demons or the magical means such as wearing of different amulets. This was coupled with empirical knowledge of variety of vegetable drugs. Ayurveda, the science of life, is the most comprehensive holistic system of healing known. This ancient healing science of India is meant to reintroduce modern man of walking with naked feet through life to come back into contact with nature. The science of life is not unrelated to Vedic literature. *Atharvaveda* is regarded as the original source of medical science. The great

Susruta has himself admitted this – *Ayurvedam namopangamatharvavedasya*[7] – that Ayurveda is an accessory to *Atharvaveda*. *Bhava-Prakasa* also endorses this view.[8]

Now, let us examine the causes of venereal diseases (VDs) and sexually transmitted diseases (STDs) prevalent in our society. Many of the venereal and sexually transmitted diseases are "imported" from the West. During past two to three decades, western world has shown increased tendency to publicise and commercialise sex and sexual acts. New techniques and Viagra like stimulants have entered most of the bedrooms and households to help achieve more and more enjoyment. As a result, sex is no more an individual affair – rather it has become a general and collective act. More a tendency spreads, more it becomes wide, powerful and decontrolled. First we use things, later things start using us. Imitating West, we too are not far behind. Young minds are drowned neck-deep in the ocean of sexuality. There is nothing but sex and sexual activities everywhere in the minds of youths, irrespective of their age and eligibility. In this unending quest for quenching the physical thirst, we have imported perverted sexual activities. It seems that the state of anarchy and promiscuity has reached a full circle. Irony is that while whole of the West which is fed up with its own civilisational artificialities is finding solace and peace in Indian traditional science of life and meditational techniques in particular, and Indian way of life in general, we on the other hand, are following their ignoble and disastrous notions as well as professing them to be imitable. Right was Mark Twain in saying that it is very difficult to make a prophecy specially when it belongs to future. The concepts of "live-in partnership", "wife swapping" and "wife swinging" has already intruded our Indian society. Dr. David Delwin, in his book *How to improve your sex-life*, makes an alarming prophecy:[9] "Two more activities which have increased greatly in recent years are 'wife swapping' and 'swinging' (which really means a more promiscuous form of wife swapping with contacts being made through magazines, newspapers, or parties). I suppose, its inevitable that more and more people will go in for wife swapping".

Our ancient seers and spiritual leaders have been true scientists and fortune-tellers who, keeping in view these perversions and fornications, emphasised the importance of celibacy and ethical values. Besides medicinal prescriptions, no other cultural tradition has emphasised the importance of celibacy and ethical values as Indian culture and tradition has. Ancient seers considered deviations from ethical values or set code of conduct, the root cause of all types of maladies. We have a glimpse of this adherence to moral values in this famous line from the scripture:

Astadasapuranesu Vyasasya Vacanadvayam
Paropakarah Punyaya Papaya Parapidanam.

Since adherence to moral and ethical values absolve us from miseries, the Indian concept of moral values needs special attention. In modern society, the value traditionally set upon chastity is in conflict with the more recent ideas of independence, freedom from supervision and equal rights for both sexes. Moral and cultural values have been relaxed. Immoral conduct leads to sheer wastage of *Prana*, the life energy. This also gives birth to emotional turbulence which causes many disruptive complexes within human beings. In the name of modernity and freedom, moral restrictions and bindings are being questioned and sidelined in many ways. These age-old, time-tested bindings are being labeled as rubbish and retrogressive. But its ill-effects are not hidden now.

The another very important element of Indian culture and tradition emphasised repeatedly by rishis and omniscient seers is continence (*Brahmacharya*) abiding which many sex-generated or sexually transmitted diseases can be avoided. Our tradition has never neglected or negated sex or sexual activities because it is one of the four supreme goals (*Purusharthas*) of life. Our scriptural injunctions only stress its regularisation and proper channelisation. Had this not been the case, Vatsayan would not have created his world-over accepted masterpiece the *Kamasutra* or the speaking carvings on the walls of Khajuraho would not have appeared. Our unique marriage system is a glaring example of according sanctity and sanction to sexual act.

This institution of marriage is generally an unbreakable bond which must have come into being just to avoid the extant sexual promiscuity and anarchy in the society in the distant past. Between married life, sexual act and continence there lies no paradox because a married person whether male or female having firm fidelity towards each other is said to be *Brahmachari* in Indian context. The purpose of propagating continence is to associate *Kama* with *Dharma*, to establish its physical and celestial value. In the *Bhagvadgita* Lord Krishna proclaims[10]: "Arjuna! of the mighty, I am the might, free from passion and desire; in beings I am the sexual desire not conflicting virtue or scriptural injunctions". In the tenth chapter again the lord says[11]: "I am the sexual desire which leads to procreation as enjoined by the scriptures" – such is the sanctity accorded to the purpose of sex throughout our scriptures. This also evinces the very purpose of the institution of marriage.

Let us have a look at the concept of celibacy or continence. The great Patanjali in his magnum opus *The Yoga Sutra* has enlisted "abstinence from incontinence" among five abstentions (yama), by the acquisition of which the yogi increases his unhindered qualities.[12] As soon as continence is established, vigour and energy is acquired. Energy is power, which if stored increases qualities – *Brahmacaryapratisthayam Viryalabhah.* Thus, it is a well substantiated fact that by the power of *Brahmacarya*, one can stay healthy, get rid of ailments, develop physical strength and mental abilities to achieve higher goals in life.

Since this discourse is centred on venereal diseases (VDs) and STDs, mention of some very common diseases is a must. It is an established fact that over-indulgence, abnormality, lack of self-control and innovations for increased enjoyment in sexual activities lead to many sexual diseases. Having sex with unfamiliar sex partners doubles the risk. This view has been supported by the *Ayurvedic* text, *Bhava Prakasa* as follows[13]: "over-indulgence in sexual activities beget acute pain, cough, fever, bronchitis, leanness, anaemia and feebleness". On the contrary, those who follow restraints in sexual act become strong in memory, intelligence, age, health and stoutness, energy of organs, frame and physical strength combined with delayed aging.[14] Seven types of ailments have been described in Ayurvedic texts:

1. (*Adibalapravrtta*) Genetic,
2. (*Janmabalapravrtta*) Congenital,
3. (*Dosabalapravrtta*) Disturbance in Homeostatis,
4. (*Samghatabalapravrtta*) Traumatic,
5. (*Kalabalapravrtta*) Seasonal,
6. (*Daivabalapravrtta*) Spiritual, and
7. (*Svabhavabalapravrtta*) Natural.

Ayurveda is based on the *Tridosa* theory of diseases. Three *Dosas* are *Vata, Pitta*, and *Kapha*. This science of life stresses the importance of hygiene and sanitation.

STDs are transmitted mostly by direct sexual contact. The factors responsible for the spread of STDs are prostitution, emotional immaturity in teenagers, sexual disharmony, changing behaviour patterns, greater tolerance in sexual behaviour, more frequent pre-marital and extra-marital inter-courses, sexual freedom and homosexuality.[15] J. E. Park and K. Park have enlisted STDs and classified them as "classical" and "other infections". Classical STDs are as follows:

1. Gonorrhoea
2. Syphilis
3. Chancroid
4. Lymphogranuloma Venereum
5. Donovanosis

Other infections include:

1. Chlamydia infections
2. Genital Herpes
3. Acute and chronic Hepatitis B
4. Mycoplasma infections
5. Trichomoniasis
6. Genital warts
7. Pelvic inflammatory diseases
8. Molluscum Contagiosum
9. Ectoparaseles

I shall not go into the details of above mentioned diseases but refer to two-three most common diseases which have long afflicted the world population and have been discussed in main Ayurvedic texts. Gonorrhoea is called *Aupasargika Puyameha* in Ayurveda and is known as *Sujak* or *Sojak* also. Others have called it *Usnavata* but it is not widely accepted. It spreads by sexual contact. The other disease which is mentioned there is Syphilis which has been designated as *Upadamsa, Phiramga, Atasaka*. Five types of Syphilis have been described[16] – *Vatika* (related to *Vata*), *Paittika* (related to bile or gall, bilious), *Slaismika* (Phlegmatic), *Sannipatika* (related to *Sannipata*) and *Raktaja* (born out of blood). 'Chancroid' or soft chancre resembles with this. Syphilis afflicts males and females both- *Strinam pumsamca Jayante Updamsasca darunah*. The famous text *Madhavanidana* describes its severity and fatality in the following line: "If not treated in time the wound spreads speedily and destroys the genitals of both males and females and the afflicted person dies".[17]

Another text, *Astanga Samgraha* describes venereal diseases called *Limgarsa*, which is akin to Granuloma GenitoEnguinale (*Guhyavaksaniyakarnarbuda*). Climatic bubo, lymphogranuloma which is marked by swelling on one thigh is designated as *Bad*. In another Tantra of Ayurveda the diseases which have been described as *Braghna* may have resemblance with it.[18] These are very brief outlines of the principal images of our ancient science, lost knowledge and old psycho-physical tradition remains yet to be discovered. Excessive perversion has generated many fatal VDs and STDs, like AIDS which are not mentioned in ancient texts because our ancestors could not envisage or predict the degree of promiscuity and perversion as is prevalent in our society.

India's legacy to the world is its culture, spiritual wisdom and ancient science and technology from Sanskrit texts. Our real wealth is an ever-flowing stream of culture and esoteric sciences and technology that can find their verification application through modern research. This requires a new generation of thinkers who appreciate the ancient wisdom and are willing to subject it to the test of time. Building a modern India with the ancient vision is the real way to move forward and gain the lost respect in the world. It is heartening to note that the present age is best suited for the synthesis between physical and spiritual demands of life. The science and the spiritualism are drawing closer. Let us conclude this discussion with the opening mantra of *Prithivi Sukta* where the *rishi* says: "The great truth, the terrible eternal law, rite, penance, prayer, and sacrifice upholds the earth. May she, the protector of our past and future, the earth, make this vast world for us".[19] Truth- the earth, the rectitude, the dedication and austerity can alone sustain the quality of life on earth.

Notes

1. *Na Jatu Kamah Kamanamupabhogena Samyati*
   Havisa Krsnavartmeva bhuya evabhivardhate
   Manusmrti, 2.94
2. *Sarvamanyatparityajya Sariramanupalayeta.*
   Tadbhave hi bhavanam Sarvabhavah Saririnam.
   Caraka Samhita Nidana 6/7
3. *Sariramadyam khalu dharmasadhnam.*
   Kumara Sambhavam,5th Canto
4. *Nagari nagrasyeva rathasyeva rathi yatha.*
   Svasarirasya medhavi Krtyesvavahito bhave.
5. *Samadosah Samagnisca Samadhatumalakriyah*
   prasannatmendriyamanah Svastha ityabhidhiyate.
   Su. Su. 15.41
6. *Dharmarthakamamoksanamarogyam mulamuttamam*
   Ca. Su. 1.15
7. *Susruta*-1.1.6
8. *Atharvantargatam Samyagayurvedam Ca labdhavan*
   Bhava Prakasa.1.58
9. pp.171
10. *Balam balavatam caham Kamaragavivarjitam*
    dharmaviruddha bhutesu Kamosmi bharatarsabha
    Bhagvadgita. 7.11
11. *Ayudhanamaham Vajram dhenunamasmi Kamadhuk*
    Prajanascasmi Kandarpah Sarpanamasmi Vasukih
    ibid, 10.28
12. *Brahmacaryapratisthayam Viryalabhah.*
    Patanjala Yogasutra 2.38
13. *Sulakasa Jvarasvasa Karsyam Pandvalayaksayah*
    Ativyavayajjayante rogascaksepakdayah.
    Bhava Prakasa, 5.113
14. *Smrtimedhayurarogya pustindriya yasobalaih.*
    Adhikamandajaraso bhavanti strisu samyatah
    ibid, 7.75

15. Text of Preventive and Social Medicine (1985), J.E.Park and K. Park, pp 362-363
16. *Pancavidhastribhirdosaih prthak Samastairasrja ca*

    Su. Ni. A-12
17. *Samjatamatre na karoti mudhah*

    Kriyam naro yo visaye prasaktah.

    Kalena Sothakrmidahapakairvisirnasisno mriyate sa tena.

    Madhavanidana
18. *Atyabhisyandigurvannasevanannicayangatah. Karoti granthivachhotham doso vanksanasandhisu. Jvarasulangasadadyam tam bradhnamiti nirdiseta.*
19. *Satyam brhadrtamugram diksa tapo brahmayajnah prthivim dharayanti. Sa no bhutasya bhavyasya patnyurum lokam prithivi nah krnotu.*

    Atharvaveda, Prithivi Sukta-1

III

Health Expenditure and Insurance

14

Health Seeking Behaviour and Health Expenditure in Tribal Areas of Rajasthan

Results for Policy Initiatives

P.R. Sodani

Overall health spending in India is estimated at 4.5 per cent of GDP, which is less than the average of 5.6 per cent for low- and middle-income countries. India also has one of the highest proportions of private health financing in the world, about 82 per cent. Only five countries (Cambodia, the Democratic Republic of Congo, Georgia, Myanmar, and Sierra Leone) have a higher dependence on private health financing (WHO, 2000a). The low spending and the dominance of private sources of financing make India unique (World Bank, 2000).

In many developing countries, governments are facing increasing pressure to improve the efficiency and financial viability of health service delivery system, particularly in the light of renewed commitments to improve the living conditions of the poor (World Bank, 1993). The case of India provides an excellent example, where almost all the state governments are facing this challenge. The situation is further grim in special population groups, especially tribal ones. They live under poor socio-economic conditions, and divergent cultural and behavioural practices. These tribal groups have limited access to health care. The challenge is therefore relatively greater in states where the proportion of tribal population is high. The case of Rajasthan provides an excellent example.

However, Rajasthan with a distinct culture, social customs, and values ranks below the national average on many health indicators. It, therefore, needs a distinct state-specific approach to improve the efficiency and financial viability of the health sector. In this background, formulation of health policies and programmes requires a better understanding of health care seeking behaviour and expenditure by households on treatment.

To improve the health status of the people of Rajasthan, the state government has initiated a number of policy reforms including the drafting of the Health Vision for Rajasthan 2025. However, more needs to be known about the household's role in financing health care. Only a few studies have investigated the level and distribution of household health expenditure in India (Duggal and Amin, 1989; George 1997; Hotchkiss, et al., 2000; NSSO 1992; NCAER, 1992; Sodani 1997; Sodani and Gupta, 1998; Bhatia and Cleland, 2001). The objectives of the paper are to understand morbidity profile, health care seeking behaviour, utilisation of health care services, household health care expenditure, and to investigate factors affecting household health care expenditure and discuss policy implications to design and implement health sector reforms.

Data and Methodology

The data used in this analysis comes from the doctoral research carried out by the author at the Department of Economics, MLS University, Udaipur (Sodani, 1997). This household survey collected information from a representative sample of 450 households, 225 from rural areas and 225 from urban areas of three districts (Banswara, Dungarpur and Udaipur) dominated by Scheduled Tribe population. The Tribal-Sub Plan (TSP) region of Rajasthan State is mainly comprised of these three districts. The data was collected during the months of June-August 1996. It was a one-time survey and therefore could not reflect the seasonal variations in the morbidity pattern. Only those households were selected where any family member had experienced an event of ill-health during the reference period (last 12 weeks from the date of survey) for which a treatment was sought. Untreated illnesses were not included in the study.

Results and Discussions

Choice for Source of Health Care

There are various types of health care facilities available for the treatment of illnesses in the area. The available health care facilities have been divided into the following five categories, i.e., public, private, traditional practitioners, chemists' shops, and family/friends, for the purpose of analysis. Public facility, included all the government-run health care institutions irrespective of the system of medicines. Private facility, included all the allopathic private hospitals, dispensaries and clinics run by charitable institutions, non-governmental organisations, and individual practitioners. Besides, medical or para-medical personnel giving treatment and collecting fees are also included in this category. Traditional practitioners included folk healers, registered medical practitioners (non-allopathic), herbalists, *vaidyas, hakims, bhagats,* etc. Chemists' shops, included the treatment taken directly by approaching a chemist's shop without consulting any health care provider. Family/friends, included measures taken for health care by family members, relatives, friends, and self at the household level with home remedies. Only treated cases were analysed here.

Table 14.1
Percentage Distribution of Sick Individuals by Choice of Source of Care in Rural and Urban Areas of Rajasthan

Type of Health Care Facility	*Rural Area*	*Urban Area*
Public facility	27.3	45.1
Private facility	20.3	30.2
Traditional practitioners	50.7	18.0
Chemists' shops	1.4	6.1
Family/self	0.3	0.6
Total sample	355.0	295.0

In rural areas, the most commonly approached source of care is traditional practitioners (50.7%) while in the urban areas it is public health facility (45.1%). The percentage of illness episodes for which medicines have been directly purchased from medical shops works out to be 1.4 for the rural population and 6.1 for the urban population. Seeking treatment from relatives or family members, i.e., dependence on home remedies seems very low, though the percentage is marginally higher for the urban areas (0.6) as compared to rural areas (0.3).

The traditional practitioners and the private sector seem to play an important role in providing health care in the study areas. The major implications are that efforts are needed to encourage public-private partnership in the current context. The private formal and non-formal sectors need to be tapped for better services in the tribal areas.

Health Care Expenditure by Households

The total health care expenditure per illness episode is the sum of direct and indirect costs incurred to recover from the sickness episode during the reference period. Direct cost, includes expenses incurred on providers' fees, medicines, diagnostic tests, hospitalisation charges, and expenses related to surgery. Indirect costs, includes expenses associated with the treatment. It includes expenses incurred on transport, food/stay arrangements during the course of the treatment, and tips given to get access to any person/facility at any level for getting better care. Also, expenses incurred for temple offerings, *pooja (prasad, agarbatti,* etc.) and similar religious events carried out for the sole purpose of alleviating the suffering of the sick person are also part of indirect cost. Then, there are opportunity costs, for example, loss of earnings to the sick individual and the accompanying person were added to indirect cost category.

Table 14.2

Average Household Health Care Expenditure per Illness Episode in Rural and Urban Areas of Rajasthan

Average Health Care Expenditure	*Amount (Rs)*	
	Rural	*Urban*
By nature of illness		
All type of illnesses (acute and chronic)	931.7	610.8
Acute illnesses	714.3	465.6
Chronic illnesses	1817.1	1655.5
By source of care		
Public health facility	621.1	304.4
Private health facility	2051.0	1384.8
Traditional practitioners	679.2	293.1
Chemist's shops	13.0	230.0
Family/friends	116.4	26.1

There was a substantial rural-urban differential in the average expenditure per illness episode during the reference period of 12 weeks (Table 14.2). On an average, rural people incurred an expenditure of Rs 931.7 per illness episode, while the urban people incurred Rs 610.8. Rural people spent one and a half times more on treatment of illness than urban people, taking acute and chronic illnesses together. However, this differential was more pronounced for acute illnesses (1.5 times) as compared to chronic illnesses (1.09 times).

As expected, the study revealed that average expenditure per illness episode was higher for chronic illnesses compared to acute illnesses. People, both in rural and urban areas, spent more on treatment of chronic illness compared to acute illness. Higher expenditures on chronic illnesses are mainly due to the nature of illnesses and their contained treatment. The rural people spent 2.5 times more on the treatment of chronic illness than on the treatment of acute illness, whereas urban people spent four times higher for treatment of chronic illnesses. One possible reason might be that the treatment of acute illnesses is relatively less expensive than the treatment of chronic illnesses in urban areas compared to rural areas. The people in rural areas suffered more even for acute illnesses. People in rural areas mostly belonged to scheduled tribal category and because of their socio-economic and cultural difference; they perceived illness in a different manner. They usually approach health facility later when the disease becomes aggravated, causing frequent visits for consultation. They believe in performing rituals for early relief from the illness.

People in rural areas spent more on treatment irrespective of the type of the facility used compared to urban areas (Table 14.2). As expected, private health facility is more expensive than any other source of care including the public facility. People spent 3.3 and 4.5 times more, when private health facility was utilised as compared to the public health facility in rural and urban areas respectively. Both in rural and urban areas, traditional practitioners are much less expensive source of care compared to private health facilities. The average health care expenditure was considerably lower for illnesses for which medicines were purchased directly from the medical shops.

The result of the study clearly indicates that the so-called "free" government health facility is no longer "free" to the household, it definitely costs to the household. Individuals who seek health care from public health system incur substantial monetary costs. The public care is associated with substantial out-of-pocket costs suggests that many public consultations involves purchasing drugs and services in the private sector.

Table 14.3

Household Health Care Expenditure Per Illness Episode by Direct/Indirect Expense Category in Rural and Urban Areas of Rajasthan

Expense Category	*Rural*		*Urban*	
	Amount (Rs)	*Per cent*	*Amount (Rs)*	*Per cent*
Direct expenditure	555.1	59.6	386.5	63.3
Indirect expenditure	376.6	40.4	224.3	36.7
Total	931.7	100.0	610.8	100.0

Table 14.3 depicts that direct health expenditure accounted for about two-thirds of the total health expenditure. This was higher in urban areas. The direct expenses accounted for 63.3 per cent in the urban areas and 59.6 per cent in the rural areas. This is probably because in the rural areas the financial burden on households is more because of special diet, opportunity costs compared to urban areas. This can be explained by the analysis presented in Table 14.4.

Table 14.4 shows the break-up of total health care expenditure by various components for the rural and urban areas separately. The components included providers' fee, medicines, test charges, hospitalisation fees, surgery, special diet, transportation, accompanying persons, tips, rituals, monetary loss of earnings to patient due to illness and loss of earnings to accompanying persons for providing support/company to the ill person during the course of treatment. The total health care expenditure is sum total of expenses incurred for treatment on all components.

Table 14.4
Break-up of Household Health Care Expenditure Per Illness Episode in Rural and Urban Areas of Rajasthan

Components	*Rural*		*Urban*	
	Amount (Rs)	*Per cent*	*Amount (Rs)*	*Per cent*
Doctor's/provider's fee	86.4	9.3	52.1	8.5
Medicine	409.6	43.9	279.6	46.0
Test charges	34.6	3.7	31.6	5.2
Hospital fee	8.0	0.9	11.1	1.8
Surgery	16.3	1.8	11.8	1.9
Special diet	51.7	5.5	6.7	1.1
Transport	71.6	7.7	94.5	15.5
Accompanying person	68.0	7.3	47.9	7.8
Tips	1.4	0.2	0.08	0.01
Rituals	1.5	0.2	0.2	0.03
Loss of earning to sick person	105.7	11.3	53.2	8.7
Loss of earning to accompanying person	76.5	8.2	21.5	3.5
Total	931.7	100.0	610.8	100.0

Analysis shows that rural people spent 1.6 times more amounts on providers' fee and 1.5 times more amounts on medicines per illness episode compared to urban people. These two items mainly accounted for a major share of direct expenses, compared to urban areas. Rural people incurred seven times more expenses on special diet for sick person compared to the urban people. This is because of the perception they have regarding special diet, i.e., for example in case of taking medicine with milk, the milk here may be considered as special diet in rural areas but not in urban areas.

Again, the expenses incurred on accompanying person is also more in rural area because of the fact that sick person is generally accompanied by two-three persons, but this is not the case in urban area. Rural people spent 1.4 times more on accompanying persons, as in rural areas the sick individual is attended by more people than in urban areas. The wage loss is also experienced more by the rural people as around 2 times in case of patients' wage loss and 3.5 times in case of accompanying persons' wage loss compared to urban people.

Factors Affecting Household Health Care Expenditure

Sodani (1999) has discussed in detail the determinants of the demand for health care by taking health expenditure as the dependent variable. The results are drawn by formulating demand for health care in rural and urban areas of the TSP region. The readers are encouraged to see Sodani (1999) for further statistical analysis. Here, the important variables affecting the household health care expenditure are discussed based on simple statistics only.

Time Gap between Onset of Disease and Contact with Source of Care

It was found that when the people fall sick, higher percentage of people in urban areas contact the source of care on the same day compared to rural areas (Table 14.5). In rural areas, only 9.8 per cent of the ill persons contacted the source of care on the day of the onset of illness. Even around 13 per cent of the sick individuals contact any source of care after a period of 10 days. The delayed reporting thus allowing the disease to progress to severe form, and this required frequent consultation and more treatment, which directly affected and increased health care expenditure in rural areas. Efforts are needed to educate the tribal community to report as soon as possible to the health care provider in case of sickness. This requires that the health services should be easily accessible to the tribal community to reduce their financial burden.

Table 14.5

Percentage Distribution of Sick Persons by Duration of Time-Gap between Onset of Disease and Contact with Source of Care in Rural and Urban Areas of Rajasthan

Duration (days)	*Percentage distribution of sick persons*	
	Rural	*Urban*
Same day	9.8	38.3
1-3	45.9	49.5
4-6	15.8	2.4
7-10	15.2	5.4
10+	13.3	4.4
N	355	295

Duration of Illness Episode

The second important factor affecting the household health care expenditure is the duration of illness episode. The duration of an illness episode can be considered as an indicator of the seriousness of the illness, i.e., the longer the duration, the greater its severity. However, a prompt curative intervention can moderate the period of illness. Table 14.6 depicts that in rural areas majority of sick individuals suffered a longer duration of illness compared to urban areas. The longer duration of sickness also contributes in increasing the health care expenditure. The longer the duration, the more will be the frequency of visits to providers, the longer the treatment duration which will increase both the direct and indirect expenses. Efforts are required to reduce the duration of disease/sickness in the community. Reforms need to focus on such measures, so as early treatment can be made available to the tribal community when it is required.

Table 14.6

Percentage Distribution of Sick Persons by Duration of Illness Episode in Rural and Urban Areas of Rajasthan

Duration (days)	*Percentage distribution of sick persons*	
	Rural	*Urban*
1-3	6.5	25.4
4-6	18.3	28.8
7-10	29.8	21.4
11-15	13.2	8.5
16+	32.2	15.9
Total	355.0	295.0

Visits to Source of Care

The frequency of visits to providers also contributed to increased expenditure for health care. Table 14.7 depicts that more number of sick individuals in rural areas visited more than two times compared to urban areas.

Table 14.7

Percentage Distribution of Sick Persons by Number of Visits Made to Source of Care in Rural and Urban Areas of Rajasthan

Number of visits	*Percentage distribution of sick persons*	
	Rural	*Urban*
Up to 2 times	63.4	74.9
More than 2 times	36.6	25.1
Total	355.0	295.0

Data depicted in Table 14.7 shows that ill persons in rural areas made more number of visits to source of care for seeking treatment than those of urban areas. It might be due to the fact that in the rural areas the treatment was mainly sought from traditional practitioners, which is less effective and of poor quality, becomes ultimately more costly to the rural people. Moreover, the people in the rural areas sought care late when the disease became aggravated, required more number of visits, resulting in increased financial burden to get health care.

Conclusions and Policy Implications

This paper provides insights into the health care expenditure at household level for both rural and urban segments of the tribal area of Rajasthan. The results indicate that health care expenditure indicators, as defined in the study, are simple but powerful indicators to estimate the nature and extent of direct and indirect expenditure borne by households for seeking health care. The household sector is contributing a huge amount in seeking health care. This has an important policy implication that households may be an important source of funds that can be used to improve the access and quality of care.

The analysis on household health care expenditure yields a number of interesting findings. Despite the lower availability of health care in rural areas, the rural individuals spend relatively more on health care than urban individuals. The reasons for this rural/urban differential are complex. It is possible that the quality of care at public health facilities available in rural areas is low, resulting in a higher reliance on traditional sector (although their quality is also low). Although rural households are less likely to seek care when they become ill, the prevalence of illness is higher and severity of illness is greater in rural areas than in urban areas. The severity of illness may be greater because illnesses suffered in rural areas may be more disabling or perhaps because rural households delay the use of service providers. One possible explanation for delaying modern treatment is that health care services are not readily accessible in rural areas.

The study shows that people in rural areas are dependent on the traditional practitioners for health care. The results raise the question whether the government services are properly targeted to those who are most in need (Scheduled Tribe population living in rural areas). Government claims that those who are poor and belonged to BPL (below poverty line) category are even exempted from the user charges at the public health facilities to provide them "free" care, which seems to be dream. The study suggests that there is an urgent need to design a public-private partnership policy for the health sector, since even though the government has created a network of facilities, these are still not being utilised at the optimal level. People preferred private sector for health care. The policy needs to be designed to tap the private sector resources to provide client centred quality services at low cost.

Another major finding is that major share of household health care expenditure is medicines. The share of medicines costs is around 44-46 per cent and makes it significantly the single most component for absorbing the costs in the total health care expenditure. The findings suggest that medicines are not available at the public health facilities, and that the individuals using the public health facility rely on the private market in order to purchase the medicines. The role of pharmaceuticals needs to be considered in designing a health policy. Moreover, efforts are also needed to encourage public-private partnership in provision of medicines.

How can government use the results of this analysis to formulate policies that will potentially improve health outcomes among the disadvantaged population? If the households are willing to pay for more health care services in the form of user fees and/or insurance premiums, alternative financing strategies such as community health financing may be have potential market if designed carefully. While these findings are encouraging, more research is clearly needed on how disadvantaged population group will respond to health sector reform initiatives. Reform strategies may be attempted first through pilot initiative to determine whether they result in their intended effects. If these pilots were successful, they would probably be a foundation stone to begin the health sector reform in the country on a large scale.

References

Bhatia, J.C. and J. Cleland (2001). "Health Care Seeking and Expenditure by Yound Indian Mothers in the Public and Private Sectors". *Health Policy and Planning*, Vol. 16 (1): 55-61.

Duggal, R. and S. Amin (1989). *Cost of Health Care: A Household Survey in an Indian District*. Mumbai: Foundation for Research in Community Health.

George A. (1997). *Household Health Care Expenditure in Two States: A Comparative Study of Districts in Maharashtra and Madhya Pradesh*. Pune: Foundation for Research in Community Health.

Hotchkiss, D., B. Kanjilal, S. Sharma, P.R. Sodani, G. Chakroborty. (2000). "Household Expenditure on Reproductive and Child Health Care Services in Udaipur, Rajasthan". In, *Financing Reproductive and Child Health Care in Rajasthan*. New Delhi: The Futures Group International, Policy Project, and Indian Institute of Health Management Research, Jaipur.

National Sample Survey Organization (NSSO) (1992). Morbidity and Utilization of Medical Services: NSS 42nd Round (July 1986-June 1987). *Sarvekshana*, 15 (4), April-June.

National Council of Applied Economic Research (NCAER) (1992). *Household Survey of Medical Care*. New Delhi: NCAER.

Sodani, P.R. (1997). "An Econometric Analysis of Health Care in Rajasthan (With Special Reference to TSP Region of the State)". Unpublished PhD Thesis. Udaipur: Mohan Lal Sukhadia University, Udaipur.

— (1999). "Determinants of Demand for Health Care in the Surveyed Tribal Households of Selected Three Districts of Rajasthan". *Demography India*, Vol. 28, No. 2.

Sodani P.R. and S.D. Gupta (1998). "Health Care Expenditure: Results from a Study in Tribal Areas of Rajasthan". *Margin*, Vol. 31, No. 1.

World Bank (1993). *World Development Report 1993: Investing in Health*. New Work: Oxford University Press.

— (2000). *Better Health Systems for India's Poor: Findings, Analysis and Options.* Washington D.C.

WHO (2000). "Health Systems: Improving Performance", World Health Report 2000, Geneva.

15

Micro Health Insurance

NGO Experience in Gujarat

Akash Acharya

Health status of populations is considered an important indicator of development (Sen, 1985). Theoretical work as well as empirical evidence have clearly established the positive link between good health and economic development (WHO, 2002). Today, health is increasingly being seen as a development issue, rather than just a medical one and apart from "natural sciences", health has emerged as a major area of academic interest in "social sciences". Since ill-health and poor health services are considered as major dimensions of poverty, efforts to combat poverty now lay major emphasis on role of health (World Bank, 2001). Out of the eight Millennium Development Goals (MDGs), which were adopted by 189 countries in September 2000 Millennium Summit at New York, three are directly related to health.

A longer version of this article has been published (co-authored with M. Kent Ranson) titled as "Health Care Financing for the Poor: Community-based Health Insurance Schemes in Gujarat" in *Economic and Political Weekly*, Vol. XL, No 38, pp. 4141-4150.

The burden of health care expenditure in general, and hospitalisation expenditure in particular, can be catastrophic for household finances. This is even truer for the poor where even a temporary incapacity of the breadwinner to earn due to illness can drive a family into destitution. Health care expenditure cuts poor's household budget in two ways. Not only do they have to spend a large amount of money and resources on medical care but also they are unable to earn during the period of illness. The evidence available from the NSS surveys indicates that health care expenditure is one of the fastest growing components of household consumption even among the poor. Between NSS 42nd and 52nd round, those sick but not availing treatment for financial reasons increased from 15 per cent to 24 per cent in rural areas and doubled from 10 per cent to 21 per cent in urban areas. More than 40 per cent of individuals, who are hospitalised, borrow money or sell assets to cover the cost. Almost one quarter of all Indians fall into poverty as a direct consequence of the medical expenses they pay, out-of-pocket, after being hospitalised (IHR, 2003).

Health Insurance and NGOs

This enormous financial burden could be avoided through the protection of health insurance but public as well as private health insurance companies have traditionally targeted only the urban middle and upper class. Large majority of poor people working in the informal sector remain outside the health insurance net. Interestingly, many non-governmental organisations (NGOs) in India have taken initiative in providing financial protection to poor by the provision of health insurance. Since the focus is on poor, such health insurance schemes are known as Micro Health Insurance (MHI). Some authors also use terminologies like Community-Based Health Insurance (CBHI), Community Health Insurance (CHI) and Community-Based Insurance (CBI) because of community involvement in such schemes.

Although there is a dearth of proper documentation, there are about thirteen NGOs in India that are running MHI scheme for poor (Ranson et al., 2003). Out of these, Gujarat is home to four such innovative health insurance experiments. Gujarat has a long tradition of voluntary organisations. NGOs rooted in Gandhian philosophy have covered a large field of development activity including health in the state. Gujarat has a relatively large number of voluntary initiatives for providing health services in urban as well as rural areas (Iyengar, 2000). Self-Employed Women's Association (SEWA), Tribhuvandas Foundation (TF), Aga Khan Health Services, India (AKHS,I) and Navsarjan in Gujarat have tried to provide financial protection to poor through MHI.* In this article, I have introduced these four schemes and have also tried to do some comparison and analysis.

Self-Employed Women's Association (SEWA)

SEWA is a trade union of more than 7,00,000 poor self-employed women in India working in the informal sector. It has been running one of the largest and successful micro insurance schemes since 1992 for its members. SEWA's scheme is known as Integrated Insurance Scheme (IIS), which provides life, health and asset benefits. The scheme charges a premium of Rs 100 per annum and provides hospitalisation benefits up to Rs 2000, Rs 3000 against natural death, Rs 40,000 against accidental death and Rs 10,000 against loss of occupational assets. Member can also choose to opt for a fixed deposit with SEWA Bank and interest on the deposit will go as premium. A woman member can also insure her husband and children by paying some extra premium. The scheme is operating in 11 districts of Gujarat state and in Ahmedabad city, which is SEWA's headquarter. Of late, the scheme has also been

* Recently, one more organisation (Shree Krishna Arogya Trust) has initiated a micro health insurance scheme in Kheda/Anand districts of Gujarat.

extended to other states of India. SEWA has tied-up with professional insurance companies like (LIC, OM Kotak, National Insurance Company and ICICI Lombard) for its micro insurance programme. For the health insurance component, pre-existing diseases are not included in the coverage and members have to pay out-of-pocket at the time of hospitalisation. They have to file a claim for reimbursement to VimoSEWA (vimo means insurance in Gujarati) after hospital discharge. Currently, SEWA is in process of establishing tie-ups with selected hospitals so that SEWA members can get cashless facility. Attempts are also being made for coverage of pre-existing disease. Today, SEWA's scheme is more than 1,00,000 members that makes it one of the successful models of MHI, not only in India but also at a global level.

Tribhuvandas Foundation (TF)

TF works in 638 out of 900 villages of Kheda and Anand district* of central Gujarat and does various development-oriented activities including health of women and children. TF has been named after late Tribhuvandas Patel, who was one of the pioneers of the white revolution and founder chairman of AMUL dairy. The health insurance scheme named as Sardar Patel Aarogya Mandal came into existence on January 26, 2001. Under this new scheme (TF had already been experimenting with prepayment for more than 20 years), 3 paisa per litre of milk deposited, plus Rs 26 (Rs 25 for TF membership and Rs 1 for the scheme) per year are collected as premium from each household. This 3 paisa per litre, were being collected years before the scheme was started to build a corpus, which would generate sufficient interest for premium of the scheme. Members of the milk cooperative are entitled to 100 per cent of hospitalisation expenses (excluding medicine,

* Information given at the time of field visit in 2002.

transport and other indirect cost) for the family. Members must deposit a minimum of 300 litres of milk per year and should not sell milk to competitors for availing scheme benefits. Under this scheme, members when in need, have to approach TF or any of its sub centres for referral to hospital. After getting a reference slip from the TF doctor, they can approach any of the nine approved/empanelled hospitals. All these hospitals are trust hospitals and patients can be admitted into the hospital by showing the membership card. Members do not have to incur any out-of-pocket expenditure at the time of hospitalisation. All nine hospitals send bills to the TF office on a monthly basis and they pass through the scrutiny by TF office staff. At the time of data collection in 2002, 83,000 families from 645 dairy cooperatives had already become members of the scheme.

Aga Khan Health Services, India (AKHS,I)

The Aga Khan Health Services, India (AKHS,I), a major functionary of the Aga Khan development network, is one of the most comprehensive, non-profit health care system in the developing world. In Gujarat AKHS,I is working in Sidhpur taluka of Patan district in North Gujarat and Junagadh district in Saurashtra. In the first scheme known as cooperative health care financing, AKHS,I has tied up with a dairy cooperative and the dairy cooperative deducts 3 to 5 paisa per litre of milk and in return provides Rs 30,000 to AKHS,I. Under the second scheme, known as community health fund (CHF), Rs 200 are collected as premium from each family who are not members of dairy cooperatives. Those who are members of any of the two schemes, get waiver in registration fee (which in any case is subsidised, at a cost of only Rs 2) and medical examination fees (Rs 5) as an outpatient benefit. They get 10 per cent discount in delivery charges. Members receive 20 per cent discounts in all laboratory tests. Moreover, all members who are above the age of 35 get free medical check up and Non-Communicable

Disease (NCD) screening once in a year. Females also get breast cancer screening free. AKHS,I does not provide any hospitalisation cover except in case of delivery. The community itself, through local health sector management committee, decides the premium amount. According to AKHS,I management, the highest utilisation of the scheme is through availing the 20 per cent discounts in all laboratory tests. Community perceives this benefit attractive as these tests are expensive in nature.

Navsarjan

Navsarjan, which was established in 1988, mainly works with Dalits. The main objective of the organisation is to unearth the atrocities against dalits and fight against these atrocities by providing legal assistance so that dalits can lead a life with self-respect and dignity. Today Navsarjan is working in 11 districts of Gujarat and has a team of 194 workers. Of late, Navsarjan has also started working for poor non-dalits and thus the focus is shifting from caste to class. One enthusiastic and committed worker of Navsarjan, who belongs to North Gujarat region, initiated an idea of health insurance. Navsarjan decided to buy the Mediclaim policy from New India Assurance (Sanand branch) and pay the premium. The premium of Rs 159 per member was partly subsidised by Navsarjan and benefits included hospitalisation cost upto Rs 15,000. Five panel doctors (2 orthopaedic surgeons, 1 gynecologist, 1 physician and 1 general surgeon) were approached in Patan town and it was decided that the members, in case of need, would visit them in Patan. The doctors agreed to receive payment after three months, i.e., they would provide treatment on credit. The village Navsarjan workers often accompanied members to the hospital in Patan and would help with required paper work. Around 574 individuals (51% of them were women) were covered under the scheme for one year. According to the data provided by Navsarjan, during the period of scheme operation (i.e., from 17/3/1999 to 16/3/2000), 57 claims were made. From these claims, 21 were totally rejected (rejection rate 36.8%) and in many cases full amount was not sanctioned. The average cost of hospitalisation works out to be Rs 1,423 whereas the average cost of reimbursement comes to Rs 808. The scheme was on a pilot basis for one year and was discontinued as the management felt that such a programme would require substantial administrative efforts, and health insurance was not the main focus of the organisation. Fraud by doctors including inflated bills, over prescription and unnecessary hospitalisation was also cited as a reason for termination of the scheme.

Discussion

MHI scheme have become well known in sub-Saharan African countries (Senegal, Mali, Burkina Faso, Ghana, Zaire, Democratic Republic of Congo, etc.) and now this MHI model is being replicated in developing countries of South Asia. MHI scheme run by NGOs in India and Gujarat are diverse in nature and each scheme is like a case study in itself. Some schemes have few hundred members, whereas some have few lakhs, some are run by Micro Finance Institutes (MFIs), some are run by broad development NGOs and some by health specific NGOs. Table 15.1 compares the salient features of the four schemes of Gujarat.

It can be seen from the Table 15.1 that though schemes differ to a large extent, the common thread tying all MHI schemes is the focus on poor and hence all schemes are low premium-low benefit schemes. Poor households contribute small amount of premium every year and get compensation or reimbursement if they face hospitalisation. The trend to forge partnership with professional insurance company is gaining ground. This can be a win-win situation for NGO as well as the insurance company as NGO can transfer the risk to the company and get the management expertise in running the

Table 15.1

Salient Features of NGO-run MHI Schemes in Gujarat

	Self Employed Women Association (SEWA)	*Tribhuvandas Foundation (TF)*	*Aga Khan Health Services, India (AKHS,I)*	*Navsarjan*
Year of Inception	*1992*	*2001*	*1995*	*1999*
Premium per annum	Rs 100	3 paisa per liter of milk plus Rs 1 per family	Rs 125 to Rs 200 per family, decided by the community	Rs 175 per individual but paid by Navsarjan to GIC on behalf of them
Benefit	Only inpatient care. Hospitalisation cover, plus one time payment for denture and hearing aid. Delivery benefits for fixed deposits members.	Both inpatient and outpatient care. Free hospitalization at selected referral hospitals	Only outpatient care (except in case of delivery). Discounts in user fees for primary care and free medical check-up once in a year.	Only inpatient care. Free hospitalisation up to Rs 15,000 at a particular hospital in Patan
Location	11 districts of Gujarat	Kheda/Anand district	Sidhpur taluka of Patan district in North Gujarat	Sami and Harij taluka of Patan district in North Gujarat
Status	Ongoing	Ongoing	Ongoing	Stopped in 2000

Contd...

Contd...

Target Population	Women in informal sector	Members of dairy milk cooperative	Ismailies* and of late other villagers	Dalits
Unit of membership	Individual	Family	Family	Individual
Members	1,00,000 individuals	83,000 families	(1) 311 families in four sectors of Sidhpur (2) 467 families in two sectors of Sidhpur	574 individuals
Collaboration with GIC	Yes (with NIC and ICICI Lombard)	No	No	Yes (with NIC)
Self-sufficient or not	Largely, although administrative cost is being paid by GTZ	No. Heavily subsidised by AMUL.	No statistics available	No. The scheme was partly subsidised by Navsarjan and partly by HIVOS

(* Ismailies is a community)

scheme. On the other hand, insurance company can reduce the administration cost of collecting premium from dispersed rural clients by working through an NGO.

But the important questions are: (1) whether MHI scheme are increasing the access to health care, (2) whether they have been able to provide financial protection to poor, and (3) whether such scheme are financially viable. Unfortunately, there is a dearth of proper documentation and impact assessment studies trying to answer these questions. Studies (Bennett, 1998) on sub-Saharan African schemes by Sara Bennett of London School of Hygiene and Tropical Medicine (LSHTM) claim that although they help the poor, somehow poorest of poor households are left out of the scheme. As far as the issue of financial sustainability is concerned, none of the scheme in Gujarat or in India is self-sufficient. They are supported by external donors (mostly international development agencies like GTZ, UNDP, etc.) without whom it would be difficult for them to survive. There is a trade-off between making scheme "financially sustainable" and making scheme "pro-poor". In order to make a scheme financially sustainable, premiums usually go up which makes it difficult for the poor to enrol. On the other hand, efforts to enrol more poor people results in lower premium collection which in turns affects the sustainability.

It seems that there is little interaction between state government's ministry of health and NGO-run MHI schemes. It is important that such schemes function within the existing health system and contribute towards national public health goals. This is possible if all stakeholders like international donor agencies, government's ministry of health, professional insurance companies as well NGOs interact more often and try to walk towards the path of universal coverage.

References

Acharya Akash and M. Kent Ranson (2005) "Health Care Financing for the Poor: Community-based Health Insurance Schemes in Gujarat", *Economic and Political Weekly* XL (38) pp. 4141-4150.

Bennett, S. et al. (1998) *Health Insurance Schemes for People outside Formal Sector Employment*, Division of Analysis, Research and Assessment, World Health Organization (WHO).

India Health Report (2003) Oxford University Press.

Iyenger, Sudarshan (2000) "Role of Non-Governmental Organisations in Development of Gujarat", *Economic and Political Weekly*, Vol. XXXV, Nos. 35 and 36, August 26–September 2.

Ranson M.K., Akash Acharya, N. Devedasan and Ruth Ann Fanstone (2003) *How to (or how not to) design a community-based health insurance scheme: Lessons learned from a review of India scheme*, report submitted to the World Bank.

Sen, Amartya (1985) *Commodities and Capabilities*, Amsterdam: North-Holland.

SEWA, Annual Report 2002.

TF, Annual Report 2000-2001.

World Bank (2001) *India: Raising the Sites – Better Health Systems for India's Poor: Findings, Analysis, and Options*, Health, Nutrition, and Population Series: Washington DC.

World Health Organization (2000) The World Health Report 2000, "Health Systems: Improving Performance", Geneva.

— (2002) "Macroeconomics and Health: Investing in Health for Economic Development", Geneva.

Index